Praise for Helen Moon

"As a first time mom, one of the greatest experiences at the beginning of this amazing journey has been working with Helen Moon. Her guidance takes the guesswork out of the process and allows any parent to be able to truly be present at this most joyful time. Now moms and dads everywhere can have a glimpse into the treasure trove of advice and insights from Helen."

—ELIZABETH BERKLEY LAUREN, actress

"Thanks to Helen we were able to get to know our newborn daughter in a way we never thought possible so early on, by paying close attention to her cues. Helen helped us see that we could foster and encourage the natural schedule that our daughter was forming. Helen taught us how to manage the most valuable commodity—sleep."

—JACKIE and JEFF SCHAFFER,
creators of FX's *The League*

"Being a new mom can be overwhelming and exciting and nerve wracking! Helen Moon taught me how to trust my instincts and helped me find my confidence which was the biggest gift!"

—ZOE WINKLER, daughter of Henry Winkler

"She was like the cavalry coming over the hill every afternoon."

— ANDREW McCARTHY, actor

"If Mary Poppins had an iPhone . . . her name would be Helen Moon."

— MAX MUTCHNICK,
creator of *Will and Grace*

"Helen's loving, can-do philosophy is based upon the radical, common-sense notion that consistency is comforting and that constancy is reassuring. . . . Our kids learned very young to self-sooth and today they are happy, independent, loving, and confident one-years-olds. Without her, we find ourselves constantly asking, 'What Would Helen Do?' But now, with this book, you no longer have to wonder."

— SCOTCH ELLIS LORING, actor, and
TODD HOLLAND, director and producer

"Helen's book is full of wonderful little gems of wisdom—one of my favorites is, 'count to ten.' Her method for helping babies learn to soothe themselves and sleep is gentle and loving and an absolute must for new parents—definitely in the category 'I wish I'd known' . . ."

— SANDEE PAIGE and KEVIN BROWN

CHERISH

THE

FIRST SIX WEEKS

A PLAN THAT CREATES CALM,
CONFIDENT PARENTS AND
A HAPPY, SECURE BABY

Helen Moon

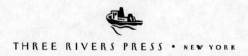

THREE RIVERS PRESS • NEW YORK

Copyright © 2013 by Helen Moon

All rights reserved.

Published in the United States by Three Rivers Press,
an imprint of the Crown Publishing Group,
a division of Random House, Inc., New York.
www.crownpublishing.com

Three Rivers Press and the Tugboat design are
registered trademarks of Random House, Inc.

Library of Congress Cataloging-in-Publication Data
Moon, Helen.
Cherish the first six weeks : a plan that creates calm, confident
parents and a happy, secure baby / Helen Moon.
p. cm.
1. Infants—Care. 2. Infants—Sleep. 3. Parenting.
4. Child rearing. I. Title.
RJ61.M7247 2013
649'.122—dc23 2012027392

ISBN 978-0-307-98727-3
eISBN 978-0-307-98728-0

Printed in the United States of America

BOOK DESIGN BY BARBARA STURMAN
ILLUSTRATIONS BY NICOLE KAUFMAN
COVER DESIGN BY MISA ERDER
COVER PHOTOGRAPH BY CHERYL ZIBISKY/GETTY IMAGES

2 4 6 8 10 9 7 5 3 1

First Edition

The book is dedicated to my Dad, Peter,
and to the memory of my Mum, Brenda,
for their constant love, support,
and encouragement always.

Also, to my two children, Baris and Olivya,
who have given me so much love and joy
and have helped me to become a better parent;
I have become a better parent advocate
because of them.

CONTENTS

CHERISH

THE

FIRST SIX WEEKS

NOTICE

• • • • • •

This book contains general information relating to the care of newborn babies. It is not intended to replace personalized medical advice, and should be used to inform patients and supplement the regular care of a pediatrician. We strongly recommend that you consult with your pediatrician about questions and concerns specific to your baby's health. The author and publisher expressly disclaim responsibility for any adverse effects that may result from the use or application of the information contained in this book.

CHAPTER 1

WHY THE FIRST SIX WEEKS ARE SO IMPORTANT

Have you ever wondered why celebrities don't seem stressed or sleep deprived, and they look so good after giving birth to their babies? In addition to the benefits of private chefs and in-home personal trainers, celebrity moms usually hire a baby specialist like me!

Now, it's your turn to learn all my inside tips for caring for your newborn. I may not be able to come to your home and guide you in person, but I can share with you all my years of baby and parenting wisdom, practical advice, and tried-and-true shortcuts. Since babies don't come with instruction manuals, the next best thing is a book that will make your baby's first six weeks as smooth and comfortable for both baby and parents as possible.

As a baby specialist and professional nanny for the past twenty-five years, I have worked closely with hundreds of families in England and the United States, and I can comfortably say that I have probably seen—and heard—it all. There's nothing like getting involved in the first six weeks of a baby's life to understand the huge impact that this short time period has on both the entire family and a child's entire life. Parents tend to be nervous, siblings are needy, and new babies need immediate and constant attention.

I can remember vividly the first day I walked into actor Andrew McCarthy's house. Neither Andrew nor his wife had had a great deal of experience with babies before, so they looked to me for guidance at every turn. We quickly established a feeding routine to benefit their new little boy, and we worked together to reset the baby's nocturnal sleep cycle, gradually teaching the baby to sleep more at night and less during the day.

Like any couple, Andrew and his wife, Carol, were full of questions: "Is he eating enough? Is it normal for him to be pooping so frequently?" And my favorite, "Is it normal to have a contented baby who is eating well and sleeping well?"

I remember vividly Andrew actually commenting

on the fact that he hadn't watched so much TV in his life, as we all sat together and watched the first series of *The Bachelor*. He was so relaxed; watching television was a pleasure, and not something he thought he would have time to do.

I think it was at this point that Andrew turned to me and said, "You need to write a book! I don't know how we would have done this without you!"

That was about ten years ago, and I am finally writing that book—for you.

In this book, I will share with you a nurturing yet practical approach to caring for babies that will show you exactly how to put your infant (or baby) on a sleeping and feeding schedule in the first week and how to help your child (or children!) sleep through the night as early as six weeks old, as well as realistic suggestions that will ensure that everyone else in the family will also get enough rest.

My plan, which I refer to as CHERISH, will show you exactly how to get your baby on a sleep and feeding schedule that will become a template for the rest of her infancy and beyond, giving her the foundation of how to sleep when she is tired, eat when she is hungry, and calm herself when she gets fussy—all of which will help her self-regulate, enabling her to thrive for the rest of her life! With these life-long skills established, you are able to rest assured that your baby is secure and happy; you, in turn, can comfortably and confidently enjoy this most precious time of your baby's life, not to mention sleep through the night yourself!

WHY SIX WEEKS?

● ● ● ● ● ●

Why are the first six weeks of a baby's life so crucial? Because in that time period it's not only possible but also absolutely crucial for parents to put into place a feeding routine and a sleeping schedule that, in essence, can help regulate your baby's internal body clock, his ability to calm himself, and other foundational aspects of physical, emotional, and social development. Does this sound too good to be true? Well, it's not. It's absolutely possible, and I'm going to show you how.

Yes, the days, weeks, and months after your baby is born are a beautiful, thrilling time period, but it's also a time when many parents panic and stop thinking for themselves. One of the first things I do when I meet a new family is reassure the parents that they already know a lot about what it takes to be good parents: we are all born with an innate understanding of what our babies need. Unfortunately, parents often

second-guess themselves, listen to others instead
of themselves, and then make themselves crazy with
worry and anxiety. These doctors, friends, family
members, and even respected experts are all well-
meaning, and often their counsel is well-founded.
But together their input often becomes a jumbled
mess of conflicting advice and a new parent in near
panic mode cannot make sense of any of it. I recently
had a famous singer-turned-fashion designer ask me
when it was okay to introduce her baby to cereal. Her
baby was more than five months old and was showing
very clear signs of needing more than just milk. But
when she asked her pediatrician if she could start to
offer her a little cereal, the pediatrician stated that if
you give a baby cereal before she is six months, she
will be prone to obesity!

The mom immediately decided that she couldn't
possibly feed her baby cereal now—even though her
instincts were probably more accurate. In this case,
with her baby only a couple of weeks away from being
six months, and clearly growing well (she was already
16 pounds), it would have been just fine to feed her
cereal a couple of weeks early.

When I was growing up in the 1970s, and even
as late as the 1980s, our parents fed babies cereal at
three months, and sometimes even earlier than that.
At that time, it was a common misconception that

putting cereal in your baby's bottle helped her sleep longer. One grandmother told me that she put cereal in her son's bottle when he was just two weeks old!

Giving cereal to newborns is dangerous, as their little digestive systems are not yet developed enough to handle more than breast milk or formula. On the other hand, I don't believe that feeding babies cereal before six months is what has created the obesity epidemic; that has arisen from lack of exercise and overeating processed food.

One of the primary characteristics of the CHERISH approach is to learn to pay attention to the needs of *your* baby, so that you can follow your instincts, think for yourself, and turn to accurate, reliable information about your baby's health when necessary.

The good news is that how you approach your baby's first weeks or months does not cause a lot of stress or require extensive thinking, but it does ask you to plan a little and stay calm a lot. What does that come down to? Be organized and don't panic! The more you are able to stay calm, the more likely you will be able to pay attention to your baby's cues, stay in tune with your newborn (or baby), and understand his needs. Is your baby hungry? Tired? Complaining because he's wet? Fussy because of gas?

Babies are not all that complicated, but when parents are sleep deprived or feel insecure about what to do, they can easily get confused, overwhelmed, or both. My approach to taking care of your baby is designed to make you feel calm, confident, and self-assured, so that you know exactly what to do; so that you and your baby can sleep through the night; and so that you won't spend twenty out of twenty-four hours each day worrying that there's something wrong with your child—or your parenting skills. I want you to be able not only to enjoy this glorious time of your new child's life but also to do so while laying down the foundation for a predictable, healthy sleeping sched-ule, good eating habits, and an overall well-adjusted child.

A LITTLE ABOUT MY TRAINING

• • • • • •

My expertise in childcare is based not only on my real-life work with all sorts of families but also on my extensive training and professional develop-ment in the areas of infant childcare, sleep, nursing, and nutrition in both the UK and the States. I have a strong educational background in childcare, hav-ing completed in 1985 the prestigious English nanny training course NNEB (Nursery Nurse Examination Board) certification. The two-year college course covered all aspects of childcare, from childbirth to seven-year-olds, including development, education, psychology, sociology, nutrition, and much, much more.

The unique aspect of this course was its invaluable amount of hands-on experience. It's one thing to be told what to do, and quite another to actually do it. We spent time on a maternity ward working with new moms, sometimes also in the delivery room. We went into a home placement to understand what it meant to be a nanny. We spent every other week in either a nursery school or an elementary school.

This hands-on form of training prepared us for what to truly expect when working with new babies and young children. During this whole process, we were continually assessed on our performance, were tested frequently on the knowledge we gained, and had numerous tasks to complete. By the time we were certified, we had acquired all the skills needed to provide excellent care of both babies and children—which is why a trained British nanny is so highly regarded.

Since I've been in the United States, I have kept up with my training and attended the University of California, Los Angeles, and completed its Certified Lactation Educator Program, just to ensure I had the knowledge to assist moms with breast-feeding.

So how does this background distinguish me

from all the other experts out there? Although I know a lot about child development and infant health issues, I am not a doctor. I'm a baby specialist. I have (and give) hands-on knowledge gained from years of taking care of babies ten to twenty-four hours a day. This experience has enabled me to understand how all children are different, how they fall into similar patterns of behavior, what they need, and what they can do without.

I've also become a parent specialist. Don't get me wrong. I think you, as the parent, will always be the person who knows your child best. However, in my twenty-five years of taking care of children, I've found that much of my time and expertise is focused on helping parents realize that they are the ones in charge and that they are the ones in the best position to respond to their babies.

For example, I recently worked for a single dad who had had a baby through surrogacy. We had a very intense first week together, as I accompanied him to the hospital and spent the first three days of his daughter's life with him, in the hospital room. I showed him all the basics, first explaining what to do and then letting him do it himself. When the baby woke at night, he was there with me, watching and learning. Then we went home and continued the routine we had established. I was so impressed to hear him explain to his parents the difference in his daughter's cries when she was just two and a half weeks old!

Another family called me when their baby was two weeks old. They were distraught and exhausted, explaining that all their baby did was cry, night and day. They had tried everything, and asked everyone they knew for advice. In two short weeks, they had attempted breast-feeding and three different types of formula. The first thing I did was to take the baby, swaddle her, and just gently calm her by talking softly and letting her know everything was going to be okay. I then turned to the parents and asked a series of questions about what they had been doing, so that I would know what bad habits were already in place. For instance, I wanted to know how she slept and where. Were they using a pacifier? Were they swaddling the baby? Why had they changed formulas? How was mom's supply of breast milk?

Then I laid out the plan for the next few weeks. We went back to breast-feeding, and I showed mom how to understand that her baby was eating enough. We gave the baby a good bath, as in their sleep deprivation they had not managed to do this. By the end of the week, we had a relaxed baby who was sleeping three to four hours during the day and four hours at night. And we had two much more confident parents, who looked to me as their savior. However, that wasn't the case: I just gave them some basic information and techniques, and showed them to trust in themselves.

As you can see from these stories of babies and their families, some of what I do is simple hand-holding until the parents feel confident and comfortable taking care of their children on their own. Sometimes this process takes two weeks; sometimes it takes just two nights. For other families, especially those who have a lot going on, managing jobs, older siblings, and other daily logistics, this can take a month or two. I will say this: most parents love having me around, but I feel most rewarded when I leave, because that means the parents have reached that place of confidence and inner calm that is so helpful when responding to babies. If I've done my job well, the family members wave good-bye, with smiles on their faces.

WHAT'S ATTACHMENT ALL ABOUT, ANYWAY?

● ● ● ● ● ●

We've all heard about the importance of attachment, that somewhat abstract yet absolutely necessary bond that needs to develop between a parent and a child (or caretaker and child), and that enables a baby to feel safe, secure, and loved. When a child's needs are met regularly, when she feels cared for and, yes, loved, she is more likely to follow a schedule and will respond well to a parent (or caregiver's) signals for a routine.

Attachment does not come from jumping up for every little squeak, or from never putting your baby down, or from sleeping with your baby all night long. Attachment develops naturally when parents stay attuned to their baby, learn how to meet his needs, and understand that it's up to them to teach the baby how to fall into a sleeping and eating schedule. Sometimes I think we should change the word *parent* to "loving teachers," and the teachers in the school should be called "educators." Then maybe more parents would understand that their role is to guide and encourage and explain to their babies and children what they need to learn. Remember, a baby is not born knowing how to comfort himself or how to regulate his sleep; it is up to you as the parent to guide your baby.

Attachment is very important because it enables a baby and young child to develop emotionally and socially, and even intellectually. Attachment is what also later enables a child to separate and become independent.

The importance of attachment cannot be overstated, but it doesn't have to be complicated. To me, attachment comes quite simply with letting yourself love and nurture your baby in a way that meets the child's needs in a consistent and calm-as-possible way.

A few years back I worked for a couple who had twins. They were so anxious about being the best parents possible that they second-guessed every little suggestion I made about establishing a feeding and sleeping schedule.

"Why should I swaddle the babies? They don't seem to like it."

"Why should we wake up the twins during the day? Isn't it better to let them sleep?" These parents came running at every little murmur that emanated from the nursery! No matter how many times I told them it's normal for babies to make a lot of noise at night, the parents wouldn't listen; they felt they were forming a stronger attachment to their babies by responding this way. They were so convinced that they had to pick the babies up every time the babies made a sound that they were completely disrupting the babies' sleep patterns. They wouldn't listen to my advice, and finally I had to walk away, as some battles just aren't worth fighting.

Consequently at seven months old, those babies still weren't sleeping through the night, so the parents brought in a sleep expert, whose advice was to put the babies in separate rooms so they wouldn't disturb each other and to let them cry themselves to sleep! Mom was incredibly emotional about doing this, but allowed it to happen. Yes, her babies learned very quickly to sleep through the night in their separate bedrooms, but all of this could have been avoided if the parents had learned to let the twins self-soothe in the beginning. It is the hardest thing in the world to hear your child crying for you because she doesn't know how to go to sleep (and hard for the baby, too!), so why put both of you through that?

HOW CAN YOU FOSTER ATTACHMENT? _____

1. Hold your baby regularly.
2. Kiss and nuzzle your baby.
3. Look into your baby's eyes when you are holding and feeding him.
4. Talk gently to your baby.
5. Respond to your baby's cries and learn to cue in to what they mean. Is your baby hungry? Wet? Tired? Gassy? These are some of the primary needs of a young baby and typically why they cry.

Of course, you can't ignore a baby's needs; on the other hand, you can't pick up your baby every time he makes a little noise. It's helpful to keep in mind that there are always going to be some days when your baby will be a little more fussy than other days. Babies will also pick up on your calmness or nervousness, your patience or impatience. By staying attuned to your baby, you are more likely to be able to distinguish between ordinary fussiness and more distress.

Babies respond best to a consistent sleeping and feeding routine. This consistency reassures new babies and makes them feel safe because their bodies and brains literally adjust to the rhythm of the routine. With a predictable schedule in place, newborns know that, after their nap and a diaper change, they will be fed. They learn to expect when they hear their nighttime music that it's time to go to sleep. These gentle cues comfort young babies, which is one of the best ways parents can show their baby love; it's also when parents can begin a lifelong bond, one that also includes time for both parents—time for sleep, time away from the baby, time to remain a happy couple, and time to be a well-balanced family.

I recently worked for a couple who had a three-year-old and a six-month-old baby. When I arrived at their home, Dad was sleeping with the three-year-old and Mom was sleeping with the six-month-old. The baby was used not only to sleeping with Mom but also to being nursed all night long! I quickly showed them how to use a reward chart to get their toddler to go to bed and sleep alone all night. After just a week, this confident three-year-old was really proud of the fact he could go to bed and sleep alone. It took Mom a little longer to allow her baby to sleep in his crib alone, but once Dad and I sat her down and told her all the benefits of having him sleep alone, she agreed to let me show her how.

We succeeded. We had to feed the baby more in the day, but he adjusted in about a week and now does very well. Mom and Dad are happily sleeping together again, and the new arrangement has done wonders for their relationship.

Calm and confident parents help create a relaxed and secure baby. A baby is very aware of its parents emotions; when you are tense and worried, it tends to make the baby tense and not feel secure. When the baby is tense, she won't relax as much as needed to release the air bubbles from eating, the burping will be a little more difficult, and the gas a little more frequent. This, in turn, will lead to a fussier baby. So it's important for the baby to feel that you are relaxed. Nature has taken this into consideration. When breastfeeding, a mother tends to feel much sleepier; a hormone is released that relaxes the mother, so she is calmer for her baby (see box, page 108). If you are not nursing, you can help calm your baby by being aware of your own state of mind. Take a couple of deep inhales and exhales. Smile. These simple actions can help your body relax while you interact with your baby.

I arrived at one family's home two weeks after their baby had been born. After two weeks of hearing their baby scream day and night, the parents were beside themselves from exhaustion and stress; they were beginning to feel that their baby was "the enemy." Mom was breast-feeding and had ample milk; in fact, the only thing that seemed to stop the baby from crying was being breast-fed. So Mom never stopped feeding her baby. Whenever she put the baby down for a nap (or a rest herself), the baby started to cry. Without hesitation, Mom would immediately pick up the baby and put her on the breast to soothe her. Of course, giving the breast would stop her baby's crying, but not for long. This constant feeding was not what the baby really needed.

It's difficult for exhausted parents to think clearly, which is why it's very important to rely on the schedule (see pages 109–113 for the Week One schedule); it will enable you to get the rest you need, and be able to cue in to exactly what your baby needs. In the case of the little one described above, when the parents took control of the baby's feeding schedule, and did not rely on reactive, on-demand feeding as the way to calm the baby, the baby calmed down. And the parents? They realized they could rely on and trust a schedule.

What does this have to do with attachment? Parents who feel calm and confident are much more likely to feel positive toward their baby. In the case of these parents, they had unwittingly given up control and had begun to feel negatively toward their little one, whom they loved so much.

A baby will instinctively bond with the people who care for him. It's a survival instinct. It's the parents who sometimes take a little longer to bond with babies. A lot of new moms bond immediately with their babies, and some dads do also. But some moms don't, and more dads take a little longer to form their bonds. This is okay; don't ever feel bad if you don't relate to your baby immediately. Becoming a parent (whether by giving birth or adopting) is an enormous transition for any person. Every day, the bond will get stronger and the joy from your baby's little achievements will warm your heart so much that there is no way you can't form a bond.

All of these ways of helping your child attach are built into my CHERISH approach. Through these simple steps, you will naturally interact with your child in a way that fosters a balanced, supportive form of interaction with your child, so that he feels and trusts in your support; then, he has the opportunity to grow and develop because he feels safe and well cared for.

You Mentioned Multiples?

I have worked with many parents of multiple births, and my approach works just as well if you have two or three babies, or more. The only difference with multiples is that you have to be even more organized. You also need to understand that you can't always calm each baby straight away; sometimes one or two of them may need to fuss a little until you can get to them. This won't harm them in any way; it will, in fact, teach them a little patience, which is much needed when you have multiples! I usually find multiples have their own, unique personalities and at least one of the babies is happier to wait while another may be more demanding. I worked with a family who had triplets, and by three months old, they were all sleeping through the night, without pacifiers and with two very proud parents!

YOU'RE IN CONTROL

● ● ● ● ● ●

Eleanor waited until she was almost thirty-eight years old to have her first child. As a lawyer, she was used to feeling confident and knowledgeable, comfortable rising to any challenges in her life. Except her newborn daughter. As soon as she and her husband came home from the hospital, Eleanor felt lost.

"Of course, I had bought about ten books on how to put your child to sleep, how to take care for your child in the best possible way—I was driving myself insane, but no tactic made sense to me. I didn't want to let my baby cry it out; I didn't want to stay awake all night holding her, either. I was so stressed that my milk was not regular, so I had trouble breast-feeding. I was a complete mess. But worst of all, I felt insecure about how to take care of my own child."

When Eleanor turned to me, her daughter Isabelle was about five weeks old; Eleanor looked as if she hadn't slept in weeks (and probably hadn't). I introduced her to CHERISH, and within two weeks mom and baby were not only on a routine with both sleeping through the night but also Eleanor was much more at ease in her new role as mom. "I think I always thought of control as something I had to force; when I figured out how to settle Isabelle down and get her on a routine, then I could relax . . . and feel more in control!"

Establishing your role as a parent is important. Many parents let their baby dictate the feeding and sleeping schedule, and so they fall into the mistake of fitting their lives into the baby's instead of the other way around. What babies want—and need—is the exact opposite. They are instinctively looking to the parent for guidance, which means giving signals that they interpret to mean you are in charge and are able to take care of them. This is true no matter how confused you may actually feel or how complicated your life may be.

As the parent, you want to gently guide your baby to fit into *your* life. Take this example: if you are a couple who tends to stay up late, instead of giving your baby his last feeding at 10:00 P.M., it may work better to do the last feeding right before you go to sleep (but no later than midnight). However, if you are an early-to-bed couple, then it makes more sense to feed your baby around 9:30 P.M., right before you like to go to sleep, knowing that your baby will probably wake up on the early side. Babies are not born knowing when to go to sleep, so it's up to you to set the timing that is most suitable to your home life.

It's also very important for parents to schedule their own sleep, especially in the early months when babies wake more frequently, needing to be fed. This strategy is best worked out with your partner, friend, or caregiver who can cover for you when you are sleeping. Moms with new babies need a lot of rest in order to stay physically and emotionally healthy and strong. If you know you will be up late or early to feed the baby, ask your partner to do the middle-of-the-night feeding. If you'd rather go to sleep at 9:00 P.M., then ask your partner to do the final feeding so you have the energy to wake up for the 4:00 or 5:00 A.M. feeding. Deciding ahead of time who will handle which feedings helps enormously to cultivate a calm home environment.

And this is true whether you are nursing or bottle-feeding. Moms who are breast-feeding can pump ahead of time (see pages 194–197 for advice on how and when to pump), so that your partner can share in the feeding.

The same is true for planning naps. During the day, rest when your baby is resting. If your partner is home, ask him to watch the baby while you sleep. You might consider asking a friend or have a temporary caregiver in place so that you can pre-schedule naps for yourself. The more you are able to take care of yourself, as well as your baby, the more everyone can trust in the routine and schedule. As you will see in the coming pages, you do have some options for establishing a routine for your baby, but most of the underlying principles are pretty straightforward.

CHERISH will show you how to manage the first, always-intense six weeks of your baby's life so that you not only give your baby the foundation to develop into a calm, well-adjusted child, by establishing a firm but loving schedule, but also make this once-in-lifetime period one you and your family can truly enjoy. Getting a baby on a sleeping and eating

Time for Yourself

Don't feel guilty about wanting some time for yourself. In fact, I encourage the families I work with to take an evening off and go out to dinner or a movie, or just have a little time alone. It's good for the soul, and you and your baby both benefit from your feeling good about yourself. It's absolutely a necessity and not an indulgence. If your baby is on a routine, then you can time it so you pop out between feeds, so you don't even have to miss out on that time. Remember, when you become a parent you don't lose the life you had— you enrich it with the wonderful addition to your family.

schedule is a dream, but it is not a mystery. It's also the single most important factor in a baby's day-to-day life, as well as for the well-being of parents and the rest of the family.

Some experts recommend an extremely strict routine for sleeping and eating; some recommend that parents respond to their babies on demand. My approach lies somewhere in the middle: it's absolutely essential that parents create a healthy, loving bond with their child, but not at the expense of meeting the needs of the child. Babies need to feel safe in order to attach, and this safety comes from having their needs met in a regular, daily way. Babies are not that complicated! When parents learn to be firm in how they guide their baby ("Now it's time to go to sleep, Johnny."), little Johnny will respond because he feels safe and knows what to expect.

All of my training and years of experience can be boiled down to one, single idea: when babies are treated with warmth and love, balanced with a firm and clear routine, they feel safe and fall naturally into a rhythm that grounds them and makes them happy.

CHAPTER 2

CHERISH:
MY APPROACH TO THE
FIRST SIX WEEKS

CHERISH is my plan of action to help your child get the best start he possibly can. It encourages good eating and sleeping habits from the beginning, which will result in a happy baby—not to mention happy, well-rested parents. It also addresses all that you need to expect during the first six weeks (and beyond), including what behaviors are normal (a lot of spitting up), what isn't normal (excessive diaper rash), and how to deal with the most common behaviors and related routines that arise during the first six weeks of your baby's life. Also covered are some of the issues that you, as a new mom and/or dad, may encounter along the way. I have laid it out in a simple, week-by-week plan so you can quickly and easily find the information you need, when you want it. Along the way, you can use my simple CHERISH philosophy, outlined below, to guide you. Let's take a look at what CHERISHing your baby is all about!

CONSISTENCY

One of the most important ways to show and teach babies and children to feel secure is to be consistent. When a baby has consistency in her life, she feels content and loved. If parents and caregivers establish consistency, children intuitively know what to expect from certain routines, which in turn decreases the chance of fussiness or difficulty with transitions. I feel it's important for parents and caregivers to be on the same page with their ideas and philosophies. However, if parents' styles do differ, as long as the parents and caregivers are consistent in their interactions with the baby, then the child will be content and learn to adjust. I've often been asked, "Why can't I get my baby to calm down and relax as quickly as you do?" My first response is always that I've done this a few more times than a first-time parent, but the real truth is that I always do the same thing to settle a baby. Babies love to bounce or be swayed a little, and with a gentle shushing, they calm down quickly. Most important, I don't get stressed about the baby being upset. The only way babies can communicate is by crying, so just remember that they are letting you know they don't feel comfortable, either physically or emotionally, at that moment and they want you to help and comfort them.

Here are some other things that you can do consistently to give your child little cues about what's happening. If you always change your baby's diaper or put a burp cloth under her chin before you feed her, she will anticipate receiving her bottle. When you sing your newborn his favorite nighttime song, he will know it's time to go to sleep soon. In short, the more parents create consistency, the more babies will cue in to signals and feel at ease and less fussy. But be careful not to create not-so-favorable habits, too! For example, if you run to your baby every time he makes a noise, then he will learn to expect your immediate attention—all the time. Then, when you don't react, he will be much more upset, and this habit will be more difficult for you and baby to break.

HAPPY HABITS

• • • • • •

Babies learn quickly, whether they are good habits or bad ones. What are the habits you should be concerned about? Little things you might find yourself doing, such as feeding your baby to make him fall asleep. "Why is this bad?" you may ask. Simply because your baby will soon become dependent on going to sleep this way, when ideally you want to teach him to fall asleep on his own.

There are a handful of easy-to-fall-into habits that can disrupt your baby's routine and your life:

- Giving your baby a pacifier at the least sign of fuss
- Rocking or holding your baby until she falls asleep and then putting her down
- Letting your baby snack on breast milk or a bottle instead of having a full feeding
- Bouncing your baby on an exercise ball or putting him in a swing or vibrating chair to help him fall asleep
- Always holding your baby and never putting her down

Giving your baby a pacifier as soon as he begins to fuss becomes a terribly difficult habit to break! To me, a pacifier stops babies from expressing themselves. Your baby could be feeling a little uncomfortable from gas; and while I admit that sucking can help, by plugging him up with a pacifier, you lose the opportunity to learn to identify his cue. Or, he could be trying to let you know that he's still hungry, maybe because of a growth spurt. Again, a pacifier will help console him, but then he isn't getting the nutrition he needs.

I once worked with a family that had triplets. I stayed with them for three weeks, then had to leave. When I returned to the household, the babies were six weeks old and all were using pacifiers to soothe themselves to sleep. This became a nightmare, as babies at that age can't keep pacifiers in their mouths, so every time they fell out, the babies awoke and cried for them. Can you image what the night was like with three babies doing that? The parents and I took the pacifiers away from each baby in succession (trying to do it all at once would have been far more difficult!), and after a few short weeks we had three babies who went to sleep unaided and didn't wake. It wasn't an easy transition, but the effort was well worth it. And the parents were thrilled to boast that they had triplets who slept through the night by three months, to the astonishment of most of their friends.

Another bad habit that is dangerously easy to fall into is lovingly rocking your little guy or bouncing him on an exercise ball until he falls asleep in your arms before you put him down. Many parents will say, "But I love rocking my baby to sleep! It's the most wonderful time in the world!" This is easy to do with a 7-pound newborn, but when he gets to be six months and 15 to 20 pounds, this becomes a back-breaking, tedious chore.

Let me share this cautionary tale. One time I was called in to help a family whose seven-month-old needed to be bounced to sleep by his nanny. It took the nanny an hour to get the child to sleep, and then she had to hold him the whole time he was asleep because the moment she put him down, he would wake up again; even when he was asleep in the nanny's arms, he wasn't sleeping deeply because he woke so quickly. I couldn't get the mom to change her ways. Mom wasn't the one who was up all night holding her baby. The mom also believed that since she was paying the nanny, it didn't really matter how her child was sleeping at night.

You're probably thinking that figuring out how to help your baby fall asleep on her own is easier said than done. There is nothing worse than getting to the end of the bottle and your baby hasn't fallen asleep, and then she won't settle down because she seems to want more milk. Just because your baby is not sleepy, that doesn't mean she is hungry. She could be gassy or just not ready to sleep yet. Immediately offering more milk quickly leads to overfeeding, which can make a baby even more gassy or cause her to spit up, waking her up anyway!

When being breast-fed, it's very common for your baby to fall asleep quickly at the breast, as there is a hormone (oxytocin) released when you nurse that relaxes you and that, in turn, makes your baby sleepy. But it is equally important to make sure your baby stays wakeful to eat enough so that she gets enough milk and will not wake because she is hungry. Babies can also quickly fall into the habit of snacking frequently, and then you end up feeding every hour or two! Breast milk is made up of two components: foremilk and hind-milk. The foremilk is the lighter, sweeter milk that comes out first, and the hind-milk is the richer milk with a higher fat content that comes out later. Babies need this fattier milk to help keep them satisfied for longer and also because the fat is important for their brain development. So if your baby is falling asleep too quickly at the breast, she is just snacking; wake her up and make sure she eats more.

You ultimately do more for your baby by letting her learn to fall asleep alone. Trust me; there is nothing better than laying your baby down to sleep,

knowing she is happy, content, and asleep, so that
you can relax, eat, or sleep yourself.

EATING AND SLEEPING

• • • • • •

To nurse or not to nurse? That is the question
many new mothers struggle with. How do you best
support your own nutrition? How do you deal with
a colicky baby who won't nap? What about the challenges, both emotional and physical, that come with
breast-feeding. And if you don't nurse, what kind of
formula should your baby have? Cow's milk? Goat's
milk? Soy? How do you stop your milk flow in a
healthy, painless way?

The answers to some of these questions are entirely personal. Some answers may emerge as you interact with your baby and get to know him. Your baby
may take the breast and love to nurse; your baby may
have trouble latching on; you may find that after one
or two weeks, nursing is just not for you. There is no
right or wrong here. You are the one to decide what
works best for you, your baby, and your family.

If you're breast-feeding, keep in mind that the
biggest and most important underlying issues with
breast-feeding are knowing when your baby is getting

enough and keeping track of how frequently your baby is peeing and pooping. You may never have discussed such things before, but believe me, this will become a hot topic very quickly after the birth of your baby!

If your baby is peeing and pooping frequently, then he is probably getting enough to eat. Eight to ten wet diapers and anywhere from two to ten poops a day are normal. Another sure sign that your baby is getting enough to eat is how long he is sleeping. Does he take a good, long two-hour nap after a feed? Then he's probably well fed. A hungry baby won't sleep so long.

Since every mother's milk comes out differently, you need to pay attention to the amount of your flow. Does your baby need to eat for twenty minutes per breast or simply five minutes? The length of time depends on how much milk you are producing and how much is coming out. (See pages 135–136 for more information on determining whether your baby is getting enough milk.) Having a full, contented baby allows for a good restful sleep.

If you are not nursing, you still need to ensure your baby gets the best nutrition possible. There are several different formulas to choose from, including organic, soy, and goat's milk. You may want to discuss what's best for your baby with your pediatrician, or do research online. Bottle-feeding your baby can be a lot less stressful, as you can clearly see how much your baby is eating. Having said this, it is also easier to overfeed your baby with a bottle if you are constantly pushing to get him to eat a little more.

I have seen so many parents label their babies as colicky (see pages 217–221 for more on this), but a lot of the time that just isn't the problem. Sometimes a baby's fussiness results simply because she is not able to burp properly. When babies cannot get rid of the gas in their upper system, they will behave similarly to colicky babies: fussy and agitated and unable to settle themselves down. It's not as easy to burp your breast-fed baby as it is a bottle-fed baby, but, yes, your breast-fed baby does need to be burped, too.

Also, there are varying degrees of gas, and if your baby has gas, it does not necessarily mean she has colic! The important thing is to establish *why* your baby is gassy. Is she overeating? Have you eaten some-thing that made *you* gassy? The general rule of thumb is that if a food makes you gassy, then it's going to have the same effect on your baby. What doesn't come up will eventually come out the other end!

There are other factors to consider, too. One reason for a baby's tummy upset (or difficulty burp-ing) may be a food intolerance. If you have a family member who is lactose, dairy, or soy intolerant, then there will be a higher risk that your baby will be lac-tose, dairy, or soy intolerant, too. This is important to know when choosing what you eat while breast-feeding or choosing a formula for your baby.

For example, one of my families had a two-week-old who had apparently cried almost nonstop for her first two weeks. I found out that the dad's side of the family had severe intolerance to lactose in both dairy and soy. Mom was breast-feeding, but the lactose in the breast milk was irritating the baby's stomach so much that the poor little thing was miserable. The fact that mom was surviving on dairy products didn't help matters, either. We cut all dairy out of mom's diet, but that didn't help enough, so we eventually switched the baby to a formula free of all lactose, dairy, and soy. The difference was like night and day. She was happy, she slept, and everyone else got some much-needed rest as well!

ROUTINE

Establishing a routine for both eating and sleeping ensures that your baby's essential needs are met and you begin to lay down the foundation for a baby who can self-soothe, sleep through the night, and adjust well. I cannot emphasize enough the impor-tance of creating and then sticking to a routine upon waking, for feeding, for napping, and then for going to sleep for the night. These points in the day and night are crucial moments when your child is looking for your guidance and when being attuned to your baby is key to understanding his cues.

You begin to establish a good routine by feeding your baby every two and a half to three hours during the first week or two, depending on how your baby responds. Some babies move from feeding every two and a half to three hours to every three hours in the course of one week. Other babies do this over the course of two or three weeks.

Babies' tummies are so small that they need to feed frequently to trigger the growth of their bodies. It's very important to feed your baby regularly and frequently during the first couple of weeks, to ensure both his health (so he can gain back the weight he lost right after birth) and that your milk production is optimal. You will also note that if you are bottle-feeding, it's a bit easier to keep your baby on a solid three-hour schedule.

Indeed, newborn babies are born nocturnal and have a tendency to want to eat more at nighttime and sleep more in the day. With a good routine, you can gently guide them away from this tendency, so they will eat better through the day and sleep better through the night.

This is where that old dictum "Never wake a sleeping baby" has to be ignored. If you don't wake your baby through the day, she will gladly sleep, but she will also be up at night! Likewise, if you feed her too frequently at night, she will tend to not want as much food in the daytime. Gentle guidance with eating times helps to reverse these nocturnal habits quickly and will help you establish a better eating and sleeping routine.

Not only does a feeding and sleeping routine help your baby's health and happiness, but it also ensures a little freedom for you. Knowing that your baby is content for the next two hours is invaluable. It means you can tell your husband you are taking a nap and not to wake you until the next feeding. It means you know you have enough time to eat and shower before it's time to feed again.

Another bonus of having your baby on a good routine is that you will learn to interpret your baby's cries and cues much more quickly. If you have just finished feeding, and you know your baby is full, yet he is not happy, then you can instantly eliminate hunger as the cause of his discomfort. If you have burped your baby well, you can eliminate upper gassiness, and the other options are now narrowed down to gas, tiredness, or a wet or poopy diaper. Understanding your baby's needs becomes less of a guessing game.

One mom thanked me endlessly when I came

along and got her baby on a routine. She had been feeding on demand, which basically meant that she never knew when her baby was going to be hungry next. What would happen if the mom had gone out to take a bit of a walk or do an errand; and during that time the baby got hungry, but she couldn't get back quickly enough? As a breast-feeding mom, she felt trapped in her home because she was the only one who could feed her baby. Once we got her baby on a routine, the mom knew how long she could go out, or how long she could sleep, or how long she had to make dinner before her baby needed to eat again. Dad also enjoyed the baby so much more, as he then had time to hold the baby without worrying about her waking up for food.

I will show you how to establish a routine, how to get back on a routine after a trip or illness, and most important, how to believe that you can stick to that routine!

INVOLVEMENT

Just as you want to help your child develop healthy attachment so she can later separate and be a self-assured, confident little person, it's important to be and stay involved in your child's world. What exactly does this mean? Sometimes it means simply talking aloud to your baby. Hearing your voice comforts a baby; she knows you are paying attention. When you spend time with your baby in an engaged, real way, she feels your engagement and your care.

Babies are not dolls! Their little brains are on fire from the minute they are alive, soaking up all sorts of signals—most of which come from you! They are natural communicators and they pay deep attention to what you say and do, and how you behave around them. Speaking to your baby in a warm, steady voice is a wonderful way to communicate with your baby, sending cues that help lay the path for the development of language. This kind of careful attunement will also help you to learn your baby's different cries and cues more quickly and easily and to bond with your baby more deeply.

Speaking clearly to your child also helps her learn how to express herself when she is older. If she understands what it means to feel tired, she will tell you "I'm tired" and not just whine or fuss. A little boy I looked after until he was nearly two was talking in full sentences before I left and could express that he was tired—well before most children can. Friends of the parents would comment on how he must be a genius, but I believe it's because his parents and I took the time to talk to him. We would simply say, "Now I'm going to change your diaper so you feel more comfortable" or "I'm going to feed you now, as I can tell you are feeling hungry." We told him we were putting on his blue sweater. If he was eating pasta, we asked if he wanted romano or parmesan cheese on top. If you start this talking from day one, it just becomes second nature and your baby will develop language quickly.

One dad told me that he felt kind of silly just talking to his baby about nothing, so I suggested he sit with his baby and read the newspaper or a book out loud. The dad was much more comfortable with this suggestion. Obviously, your baby doesn't understand every word you say in the first few weeks, but if you speak to your baby in a calm, pleasing voice, he will be happy to listen to just about anything!

Involvement is also a little more than just communicating. It's watching your child and following her cues, as well as guiding her cues. In the first few weeks, this involves knowing that when she screws up her face and pushes down with her little body, that means she's about to have a bowel movement and you need to respond by changing her diaper.

If you notice that she keeps pulling her legs up to her chest, you will soon realize that she is probably showing you she has gas. How do you respond? By rubbing her tummy, helping move her legs up and down to relieve the gas, or once she is more than a month old, giving her some gas medication.

Do you notice him *rooting* around? Would you be surprised to know that this is a sign of hunger? The more often you attune to the signals and ways babies express themselves and their needs, the more likely you will be to understand those needs and even anticipate them. This kind of interaction is key to establishing a bond with your baby.

SELF-SOOTHING

When you help your baby to learn to self-soothe, you give him the emotional tools that will last a lifetime—literally. Those children who can soothe and calm themselves will fall asleep and stay asleep, manage transitions, both big and small, with more ease, and become more grounded and peaceful—even as infants! Time and time again, I've watched parents use the elements of consistency, happy habits, eating and sleeping, routine, and involvement to lay down the foundation for their child's growing ability to self-soothe.

But I need to make something perfectly clear: teaching your child to self-soothe does not mean leaving your child to cry himself to sleep. I also do not mean ignoring your child when he's in need of attention. So, defining what I mean here is important. If your child is happy and calm, and has a clean diaper and you know he isn't close to needing to eat, but he's sleepy, put him down in his bed. You can stay by him, talk quietly, or sing him a good night song, but let him put himself quietly to sleep. If your child is not happy, then pick him up and rock him a little or burp him. Then once he is calm, put him back down again. The important thing is that you are meeting your child's needs when he cries out, but then reinforcing your guidance by putting him back down again. Consistency and repetition of this pattern will teach your child to go to sleep on his own. It can be a little time-consuming and tedious, but you will reap the rewards quickly.

One mom said to me, "But I want to hold my baby when he is sleeping, and I can't if I have to always put him down." My response to this is that you absolutely can hold him sometimes when he is sleeping, but let him put himself to sleep first, then pick him up again after. That way you both win: he gets the teaching he needs, and you get to hold your baby and love him when you want to! You will see that helping your baby develop the confidence he needs to self-soothe comes from guiding your baby gently, not feeding him every time he appears fussy and not overresponding to every situation.

HEALTH

* * * * * *

Every baby is a unique individual. Babies also have different health issues. If you have a baby with moderate to severe reflux, for example, then you will have to hold her up for longer, and in some extreme cases have her sleep in a propped up position, so you won't be able to follow my prescribed sleep routine in quite the same way. But you can still keep the feeding schedule. A baby with medical problems will obviously need to be treated according to your doctor's orders, so the routine I recommend for a healthy infant won't be able to be established until the baby is well and cleared by your pediatrician.

When you follow these steps and your baby is eating well, has learned to self-soothe, and sleeps, you will have a happy baby! It's not complicated; it's a mixture of love and gentle guidance, with a lot of consistency! I look forward to helping you through this amazing time with your new baby.

DEBUNKING MYTHS

● ● ● ● ● ●

Over the years, I have heard many a tall tale, un-corroborated "facts," and misleading myths that have caused much confusion for parents, relatives, and well-meaning friends. With that in mind, I've gathered some of my favorites to put them to rest, once and for all!

Managing Multiples

All of these steps to a consistent routine can be followed whether you have one baby or multiples. When it is time to feed one baby, you feed them all together. If you are breast-feeding, you can breast-feed two babies at the same time, but it is obviously not possible to feed three at the same time. In that case, you feed them back to back. Or, if you don't have enough milk to feed all three, you can alternate between feeding one baby by bottle and the other two by breast (or vice versa), making sure they all get equal time at the breast. Or, you can pump after each feeding so that the third baby will have pumped milk for the next feeding. The same goes for napping: you put them all down to sleep at the same time.

Quadruplets and other multiples are simply beyond the scope of this book.

1. **IF YOU DON'T HOLD OR NURSE YOUR BABY IN THE FIRST FEW HOURS AFTER DELIVERY, YOU WON'T BOND ADEQUATELY.**

Everybody's maternal bond kicks in differently. Bonding with your baby can happen instantaneously or it can take a little time to develop. I didn't see or have contact with my son for twenty-four hours after he was born, because of medical reasons. But when I did hold him for the first time, it was pure love! He nestled into me and was happy to nurse. On the other hand, I worked with a mom who stayed with her baby every precious second for the first four days in the

---

IF YOU JUST FOUND THIS BOOK . . .

If you're arriving at this book when your baby is older than six weeks, don't fret. Most, if not all, of this advice can be adapted to the age of your child, with the same results: a calm, happy baby who is settled into a reliable eating and sleeping routine. You will find highlighted boxes in Weeks Two, Three, Five, and Six, indicating what adjustments to make to your baby's schedule if you arrive to CHERISH after Week One.

hospital, but the moment she got home she suffered from severe postpartum depression and she rejected her baby for the first year (this was an extremely bad case of postpartum depression and not normal at all). Some dads take a little longer to bond with their babies, especially the first child, simply because becoming a parent is such a dramatic change in life. The reality can take a little while to sink in! The amazing thing about babies is that they will love unconditionally the people who care for them.

2. NEVER WAKE A SLEEPING BABY.

Babies are born nocturnal. They have just spent nine months in the womb, being rocked to sleep through mom's movement in the day and they wake up when mom relaxes at night. This is when mom typically feels them kicking. Once they are born, it's up to parents to gently disrupt these nocturnal habits and nudge them into being more awake during the day and sleeping at night. If you take control and gently awaken your baby to feed him at the proper hour, you can help regulate him and his schedule. There is no harm in doing this; you are teaching your baby when to sleep and when to eat. Remember: being a parent means guiding and teaching your child, and this starts from day one!

3. BABIES' CRIES ARE ALWAYS DISTINGUISHABLE.

This is something that I see parents struggle with a lot. They feel they should understand their baby's cries from the beginning, and they desperately try to interpret what their baby needs. As a consequence, they end up misinterpreting what the baby needs and possibly feeding the baby when the baby is simply sleepy and trying to settle. So don't pull your hair out trying to distinguish the differences among your baby's cries. Just know that through a routine and a little time you will understand what your baby is saying to you. When you learn to tune in to your baby's cries and other patterns of expression, you will begin naturally to discern what the baby needs.

4. NEWBORN BABIES JUST EAT AND SLEEP ALL THE TIME.

Not quite! Yes, your baby will be very sleepy, but she can also be a little restless from gas, from needing to poop, from not knowing quite how to settle, from needing to learn to sleep at night instead of during the day. The average newborn will sleep anywhere from fifteen to eighteen hours a day, and when you take into consideration the feeding and changing, there isn't a whole lot of time in between. The problem is that the sleep is in short spurts in the beginning, so it doesn't feel like the baby is asleep that much!

5. BREAST-FEEDING IS EASY.

It sure can be! And it can also be the most amazing feeling and bonding time between mother and child, which is not to say that the bonding between parent and child is less strong when you bottle-feed. But more to the point: breast-feeding doesn't always go so smoothly. The size and shape of your nipple affect how easily your baby can latch on; inverted nipples make it a little harder. Similarly, when your milk first comes in, engorgement can be quite a challenge for both mom and baby. The fullness of mom's breasts can cause her discomfort and even some pain. The hardness of her nipples at this time can make it difficult for new babies to latch on. So please don't assume that breast-feeding happens naturally; like any other skill, there is a learning process for both mom and baby. But once you have both learned the ropes, the experience is just fantastic.

6. IT'S BEST TO FEED A BABY ON DEMAND TO MAKE SURE HE OR SHE IS GETTING ENOUGH TO EAT.

Simply not true. But you can learn to know when your baby is getting enough so that you don't make yourself crazy with worry or second-guessing. The most obvious clues that your baby is eating enough are frequent wet and poopy diapers, and baby isn't waking every hour to eat again. Remember: every cry does not mean your child is hungry, so don't presume he is. The ability to settle to sleep is also an indication that your baby is content and has eaten enough.

7. IT IS GOOD TO TALK "BABY TALK" TO THE BABY.

No, no, no, no, no! I haven't quite figured out why people have a need to resort to a bizarre baby language when they come in contact with a baby. Remember that your baby will learn to talk by hearing you talk. Does she really need to learn that *baba* is not the real name for a bottle? The more clearly you talk to your baby, the more quickly your baby will learn language. Even repeating simple sounds like "Oooo" and "Aah" and overemphasizing your lip movement will help her.

8. BABIES CANNOT TALK.

Absolutely not true! Babies will try to communicate with you from day one. Their language is limited to crying initially, then to vocalizing. But that is your baby talking to you. It really is the cutest thing ever to watch them vocalize.

9. YOU SHOULD WAIT UNTIL YOUR BABY IS FOUR MONTHS OLD TO START SLEEP TRAINING.

You shouldn't be surprised to know that this myth in particular drives me crazy! I hear pediatricians giving this advice, over and over again. They tell the parents not to worry about how many times the baby wakes up at night, because when the baby is four months old, they can then just let the baby cry it out till he sleeps! But why do this when parents can gently encourage a good sleep routine and habits before this and have the baby sleeping through the night by six to twelve weeks old? Who wants to listen to a child screaming because you suddenly won't go into him when he is asking? That seems much more harsh and stressful (for parent and child!) than gentle encouragement from the beginning.

10. MY BABY DOESN'T LIKE BEING SWADDLED.

This is a common misunderstanding. Babies are born with an immature nervous system, and so they constantly startle themselves when they move. We swaddle to help control this startle reflex, so they have more restful sleep. Some babies wiggle more than others and will often squirm their way out of a swaddle if you don't wrap them securely or correctly. This doesn't mean your baby doesn't like the swaddle; it just means you have an active, healthy baby. By the time you remove the swaddle, at around four months, the baby's nervous system has matured and the startle reflex has subsided, and the baby is able to have a restful sleep without the aid of the swaddle.

11. CAN I SPOIL MY BABY IN THE FIRST SIX MONTHS?

I once read about a doctor who said you couldn't spoil your baby in the first six months, as a baby doesn't have the ability to manipulate his parents at such a young age. I had to chuckle that the concept of "spoiling your baby" implied that you had a bratty baby who screams when he doesn't get what he wants. The only sure way of spoiling a young baby is by not taking charge and by creating bad habits. So the reality is yes, you can spoil your baby in the first six months—just not the way you probably thought!

12. BREAST-FED BABIES WILL NOT SLEEP THROUGH THE NIGHT.

Simply not true. A breast-fed baby can sleep just as well at night as a bottle-fed baby. It's a common belief that, as formula is heavier and more slowly digested, a baby will sleep better. Even though sleep is related to your baby's eating well, it doesn't matter if your baby is taking breast milk or formula. The baby is simply learning how to put herself to sleep.

CHAPTER 3

GETTING READY:
WHAT TO DO BEFORE THE
BABY ARRIVES

Many of you will have picked up this book before your baby arrives. If you're like most of my families, you have spent a lot of time dreaming. Now it's time to make sure you have all the equipment and supplies that you need and prepare as much as you can before the little one is in your arms.

In this chapter you will find several lists—from diapers to bottles to breast-feeding needs and diaper ointments—that are intended to help you prepare for the arrival of your little one (or ones!). You will find questions to ask yourself and pediatricians you are considering, tips on essential products and baby gear, and information that might help you consider how you want to deliver, receive pain medicine, and fill in your birth plan.

CHOOSING YOUR PEDIATRICIAN

· · · · · ·

Often, when I am interviewed by expectant couples, I will be asked to either recommend a pediatrician or offer some advice on how best to choose a pediatrician. Obviously, there are thousands of wonderful, caring, well-educated, and highly trained pediatricians all over the country; it would be impossible, and not fair of me, to make any such personal recommendations. However, I have put together a working list of questions that I share with parents as they consider what's important for them in a doctor who will help take care of their precious little ones from birth through the next eighteen years.

Here is a list of questions to ask yourself (and the pediatrician) as you consider making a decision:

- What are the doctor's views on giving vaccines?
- What are the doctor's views on feeding? Is the doctor pro breast-feeding? Is he pro scheduling or does he believe in feeding on demand?

- How would the doctor help you if you were having problems with your baby sleeping at night?
- Do you like the doctor's style or personality? Do you feel comfortable asking her all the questions you might want to?
- Who will see you if your primary doctor is not available? Do you like the other doctors in the practice and the nurses/nurse practitioners? Do they have the same views as your primary doctor?
- With which hospital is the pediatrician affiliated? Is that hospital convenient to your home?
- If your baby is rushed to the hospital, is your pediatrician willing to come to the hospital and step in if needed? What is your pediatrician's protocol for helping your baby in the hospital? Will he visit you after delivery? Do you need to go to his office for the first appointment?
- Do you like the physical space of the doctor's office? Does it have a well-baby entrance as well as a sick-child entrance?

Consider these questions as you think about who you want to take care of your baby. You don't want to be in the position of arguing with your baby's doctor or feeling intimidated or at odds with his approach. You also want to feel that your pediatrician is invested in you and your family—that he cares enough to take time during well visits (weekly, monthly) and annual checkups as well as in more acute situations. To a good doctor, no question is a foolish question.

GETTING THE HELP YOU NEED

• • • • • •

Every parent needs help. This is when you need time to recover physically as well as to integrate your new baby into the family. Will Dad or your partner take time off? If your husband or partner is a workaholic, make him commit to time off before the baby arrives, but also be realistic and make sure you have additional help

These are questions you and your partner need to discuss before your baby arrives home:

1. Will you hire a baby nurse? A doula? Will your mother or mother-in-law or other relatives be on hand to help out? If they can't help out with the baby, can they bring food?

2. Do you have any friends who will be there for support? Can they bring you food? Will they help you with the baby?

3. Would you like someone to guide you and teach you how to feed, nurse, change, bathe, dress, and schedule your baby correctly, instead of learning through trial and error? If cost is not an issue, consider hiring a baby nurse.

Keeping Fido in Mind: Pet Adjustments

Many families forget to consider the impact of a new baby on a family pet. Have you considered, for instance, who will take care of your pet while you are in the hospital? Also, consider if your pet might need training not to jump at you or the baby. This kind of reaction to a new baby is more common for dogs than cats, and is especially a problem if you have a big dog. Dogs tend to become very protective of a new baby; indeed, I have even seen a few dogs that alert the parents or caregivers when the baby is crying. Most cats tend to be curious about a new baby, but they will initially keep their distance. However, remember that a cat likes to sleep in warm spots, so make sure your cat isn't able to get into the baby's crib.

Ask your friends who have children if they had or can recommend a baby nurse. Word-of-mouth referrals are always the best. Think about it early, as most good baby nurses get booked far in advance! You will also want to consider whether you need a baby nurse twenty-four hours a day or just at night. A night shift is usually twelve hours, from 7:00 P.M. to 7:00 A.M. or 8:00 P.M. to 8:00 A.M., for example.

WHAT YOU NEED

Here, you'll find a group of lists for everything you need to prepare for your baby's arrival. Remember, it's wise not to wait until the last minute to purchase necessary items for the nursery, especially the larger pieces of furniture, including the bassinet, crib, changing table, and rocker. I encourage you to go through the list at least a month before your due date and purchase or order what you will need well in advance of the baby's arrival.

In some cultures, families will not bring baby clothes or equipment into the house until the baby comes home. (It's considered bad luck.) However, I would recommend checking the availability of certain items before your baby is born, so you don't have to wait too long. Some stores will hold the items for you until you want them delivered or you can arrange for a friend of the family to hold them for you. Knowing what you need ahead of time, and having someone pick it up or order it for you when you have your baby, is the best thing to do.

NURSERY

1 crib *Many stores will try to sell you matching duvets or quilts for the crib. They really aren't necessary, as these are too heavy and can be a suffocation hazard.*

2 crib sheets

2 mattress pads

crib bumpers *Don't get ones that are too thick; thinner ones are now recommended (or none at all).*

1 bassinet *Not really a necessity, but nice to have if you would like the baby to sleep in another room in the day time.*

2 bassinet sheets

8 receiving blankets *For bundling or swaddling the baby. Choose a type that stretches as opposed to the plain cotton ones, which have no give in them. Also, think about the fabric: if you live in a cooler climate, you will obviously need a warmer receiving blanket. Muslin blankets are great options, as they offer warmth but also allow airflow. They also have a little stretch and give to them.*

changing pad and at least 2 covers

changing table

glider or rocker

8 lap pads *To protect you or your caregiver's lap from leakage while feeding or holding your baby.*

12 burp cloths

6 bibs

DIAPERING NEEDS

diapers *I recommend buying two packs of newborn diapers. Depending on the birth weight of your baby, they might not be in the newborn size for very long; two packs are enough for the first few days, then you can buy the size you need.*

Aquaphor ointment *One of my favorites for preventing diaper rash, to be used at every diaper change. If your baby does develop diaper rash, my favorite cream is Egyptian Magic; a less expensive brand is Nature's Baby diaper cream.*

wipes *I prefer to use just water or dry wipes on babies for the first month or two. You can also use the gauzelike pads that the hospital sends home with you, OB wipes (obstetrical toilettes), or even plain white Viva paper towels, which are exceptionally soft for a baby's skin.*

wipe warmer *The newest wipe warmers now come with their own washcloths, which can be washed and reused and are more convenient.*

diaper bin *The Diaper Genie, the Diaper Dékor, and Diaper Champ are good options for diaper dispensers. Make sure you also buy the liners that match the specific dispenser.*

CLOTHES

The following is the minimum amount of clothing that I feel is needed for a newborn one to six weeks old. However, if you live in a cooler climate and have a winter baby, you will probably want to add a few more onesies in a heavier fabric, such as brushed cotton or fleece.

6–8 onesies

4 gowns

2–4 hats

4–6 footed one-pieces, or tops and pants

3–6 pairs booties or socks

2 sweaters

3–4 T-shirts with long sleeves

FEEDING

If nursing:

breast pump, breast pads

nursing pillow

If bottle-feeding:

8 bottles *Don't buy more than four 4-ounce bottles, as your baby will grow out of this small bottle quickly. I*

*prefer Born Free, Avent, or Dr. Browns; most bottles
are BPA free now.*

4–8 nipples   *Make sure you have size 1 nipples to start,
and purchase a few size 2 nipples as well.*

bottle sterilizer   *I recommend the Avent electric
sterilizer.*

bottle drying rack

bottle brush

MEDICINES

Baby Tylenol

Mylecon or gripe water

rubbing alcohol

hydrogen peroxide

first aid kit

Neosporin

medicine dropper/syringe

gauze pads

nasal aspirator   *Bring home the blue one from the
hospital. There is a new nose cleaner called the Nose
Frida, or snot sucker. It's a great alternative to the
aspirator.*

cold mist vaporizer/humidifier

thermometer (rectal or ear)

Managing Multiples and Car Seats

I recently worked with a family who had triplets. Sorting out the best type of car seat to buy and the right configuration and placement for the car seats in their car was a daunting task. Were they better off having a baby car seat that they could take in and out of the car (bearing in mind that's three car seats to carry) or would they be better off with fixed car seats and take the babies out with a stroller?

The family already had the baby car seats, so we started by bringing the babies in and out of the car in their seats. This was a chore. We then switched to leaving the seats in the car and carrying the babies out to them, but this always required two people. I then suggested we put the babies in their stroller and push them out to the car, which meant that one person could get all three of them in the car. This ultimately made life a little easier. As the baby car seats take up more space than the regular car seats, we then figured out that it would be best to switch to the convertible car seat that gave them more maneuverability in the car.

TOILETRIES _____

shampoo and body wash *I like the California Baby products.*

baby lotion

baby oil

baby cornstarch powder

petroleum jelly *Only if you are having a boy who will be circumcised.*

sterile cotton balls

baby nail scissors or clippers

baby brush and comb

BATHING

bathtub *Look for one with a hammock or support for the baby.*

contoured sponge *For the tub, but also good for sponge-bathing before the cord falls off.*

2 hooded terry cloth towels

8 washcloths

GEAR

mobile *When choosing a mobile, look for one that is colorful and has music and movement. Remember, what is cute to you isn't always appealing to your baby; babies tend to like sharp, contrasting colors, not pastels!*

rear-facing infant car seat *You may benefit from checking* Consumer Reports *to research the best and safest brands available.*

stroller

sling or carrier *I love the Moby wrap, as well as the Baby Bjorn, when babies are small; the Ergo Baby carrier is very popular when babies get a bit bigger.*

baby monitor *Some have two receivers, so you can leave one in your bedroom and keep the other wherever it's convenient.*

bouncy seat *One for each baby, if you have multiples.*

Choosing a Stroller that's Right for You

As much as choosing a stroller is a matter of personal taste and your wallet, you also want to bear in mind where you live. If you are in a city, you probably want a stroller that is smaller and lighter so that it is both easy to get in and out of a car and good for general walking. Consider one with a bassinet or convertible seat, so your baby can get out more at a younger age. If you are in the country, you may need a more rugged stroller with bigger wheels.

You want to think about the weight of the stroller and how far it reclines. Safety is important. Is the stroller stable with and without a diaper bag? Does it have a five-point harness? Make sure to check the height of the handles; taller parents may need adjustable handles so they don't have to stoop. How easily the stroller folds and how much trunk space it takes (if you have a car) are also important considerations.

1 Boppy cushion *Or other baby support cushion that can also be used while feeding.*

SETTING UP THE BABY'S ROOM

'•••••

've always been a bit surprised at how some parents set up a baby's room willy-nilly, without enough thought about what's best for the parents and the baby. Here's an example of how to set up your nursery.

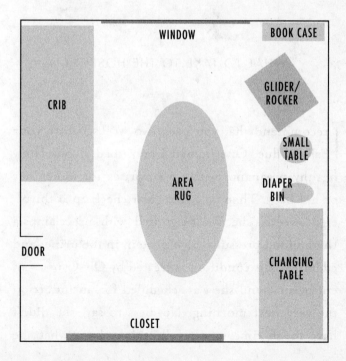

WINDOW

BOOK CASE

CRIB

GLIDER/
ROCKER

SMALL
TABLE

AREA
RUG

DIAPER
BIN

DOOR

CHANGING
TABLE

CLOSET

Remember:
- Never place the crib or the changing table right under a window.
- Always make sure the diaper bin is next to the changing table.
- Always have a small table beside your glider/ rocker for a small clock, cups, bottles— anything you need to have close at hand.
- You should be able to reach diapers, supplies, clothes, and blankets without walking away from your baby while he is on the changing table.

WHAT TO TAKE TO THE HOSPITAL

I recommend that you pack two weeks before your baby is due. One woman I know had a completely healthy pregnancy with no surprises for either her or her baby. Then, at her regular check up at thirty-eight weeks, she was diagnosed with preeclampsia (high blood pressure, high protein in the urine, and edema). This condition is treated by Ob-Gyns as an emergency, and she was scheduled for an induction the very next morning. Needless to say, she didn't have much time to carefully think about what she wanted to bring to the hospital! Everything worked out fine for this woman, and she and her baby were happy and healthy. But she did come home to a nursery that was not at all ready for her and her new baby daughter.

So let me make a suggestion: pack your bag well in advance!

You will need:
✔ cash for cab or parking
✔ watch with a second hand so you can time the contractions
✔ notebook and pen to record contractions
✔ insurance card/information
✔ toothbrush, toothpaste, mouthwash
✔ slippers
✔ makeup (keep it simple!)
✔ soap or body wash, deodorant, body lotion, shampoo, conditioner
✔ hairbrush
✔ sugarless lollipops to keep your mouth moist
✔ heavy socks for cold feet
✔ snack foods, such as nuts or fruit bars, bag of almonds, or trail mix
✔ address book or contact list in your mobile or cell phone so you remember who to call or contact!

- ✔ a robe and 2 or 3 washable nightgowns if you don't want to use a hospital gown
- ✔ eyeglasses or contacts, if needed
- ✔ CD player or iPod with favorite music for relaxing
- ✔ outfit for coming home
- ✔ shopping bags for bringing home gifts
- ✔ outfit for baby to go home in: undershirt, stretchy or gown, socks and/or booties, receiving blanket, bunting or heavy blanket in cold weather
- ✔ infant car seat

DECISIONS, DECISIONS: MENTAL PREPARATIONS FOR GIVING BIRTH

Once you're at the hospital and find yourself in the middle of the drama that is childbirth, you may not think as clearly as you might wish. With that in mind, I have gathered here some information that may help you prepare for the momentous day. It's helpful to do a little mental preparation for what to expect in the minutes, hours, and days after you give birth. By the way, this advice applies if you are adopting or having a child by surrogate, or whether your baby is brand-new or a little older.

BIRTHING CHOICES

Many first-time parents benefit from attending a birthing class. These classes teach techniques for coping with labor, including controlled breathing. They also provide detailed information about what to expect in the hospital—from what to bring, to when to ask for an epidural, to how to make sure your baby is brought to you quickly after delivery. In particular, these classes give an overview of the most widely used methods of childbirth preparation.

• **Active birth** Not a new method at all, *active birth* is a way of describing how women the world over have always behaved during labor and birth. In an active birth, the mother herself is in control of her body. She moves and changes position freely, as opposed to an *actively managed birth*, where the medical personnel control the birth process and she is a passive patient. An active birth is one in which the mother's own instinctual and natural resources take the lead and the last resort is medical intervention.

• **Lamaze technique** A prepared childbirth method developed in the 1940s by French obstetrician Dr.

Fernand Lamaze, the Lamaze Technique is an alternative to the use of medical intervention during labor. Dr. Lamaze was influenced by Soviet childbirth practices, which involved breathing and relaxation techniques under the supervision of a *monitrice,* or midwife. Modern Lamaze childbirth classes teach expectant mothers the breathing techniques and often other ways to work with the labor process to reduce the pain often associated with childbirth, such as using hot and cold packs, changing positions, sitting on a "birthing ball" to remain in an upright position, and using an orgasm to induce or hasten labor.

• **Bradley Method** Stressing the importance of "healthy baby, healthy mother, and healthy families," the Bradley Method attracts couples who are committed to taking responsibility for both the preparation and the birth of their baby. Couples train together in a twelve-week series of classes that emphasize natural childbirth instruction, relaxation techniques, using partners as coaches, and creating natural birth plans (i.e., no medication).

• **Hypnobirthing** A birthing technique developed by Marie Mongan, a hypnotherapist, hypnobirthing is sometimes referred to as the *Mongan Method.* It is based on techniques used to relax and focus attention away from the pain of labor. Ms. Mongan's program (which is certified by the HypnoBirthing Institute) was originally based on the work of Dr. Grantly Dick-Read, a British obstetrician who first introduced the concept of natural childbirth in the 1920s. The method teaches that, in the absence of fear and tension, severe pain does not have to be an accompaniment of labor. The mother learns how the birthing muscles work in harmony and how to use her natural birthing instincts for a calm, serene, and comfortable birthing.

How you choose to give birth is a personal decision, and one you make with your partner and doctor. No one way is best. However, become familiar with the different approaches so you can be more comfortable with your decision. Many Ob-Gyns and hospitals, and most midwives and birthing centers, will ask you to fill out a *birth plan* before delivery. This collection of questions will help you review your birthing options and other choices related to how you wish to deliver, including pain medication. Take advantage of this step to review your decisions and thoughts about how you wish to deliver, and whether or not you would like your baby brought to you immediately or let the nurses take the baby to the nursery so you can get some rest. Of course, you can always change your mind, but having given these questions some forethought may help reassure you.

You're in Control: What to Know About Pain Medicines

Women have used nonpharmacologic pain-relief measures to assuage labor pain for centuries. Some of these techniques include paced breathing, change of position, massage or therapeutic touch, visualization, hydrotherapy (bath, shower, or Jacuzzi), local application of heat or cold compress, and music for relaxation.

Women also rely on medicines to manage the pain of labor, including physician-prescribed narcotics, epidurals, and sedatives. Again, the choice of how you manage your labor and delivery, and the use of medicine, is entirely personal, but a decision you should be thinking about in advance of delivery.

After delivery, a breast-feeding mother's biggest concern is, "Should I take the painkillers and how will they affect my baby?" Although women are known to have higher levels of pain tolerance than most men, is this really a time to test that theory? No, is my answer! My golden rule is "Everything in moderation."

If you are so uncomfortable, you are doing yourself and your baby a disservice. You will become exhausted more quickly, and will find it harder to attend to your baby's needs. So take enough medication to lessen the pain so you can relax and rest. If you have had a c-section, you will definitely need medication! But don't overdo it, as a small amount of these medications do get into your milk supply. These tiny amounts have a small effect on your baby, making her a little sleepier than usual, which isn't a terrible thing in the first few days.

Birth Planning Worksheet

NAME: _____

DATE: _____

n   1. I have prepared myself for a birth that is as safe and healthy as possible and I prefer that medical interventions be used as a last resort, if at all.

n   2. I plan to be actively involved in all decisions related to my labor and birth and request clear and open communication between myself and all medical support staff. While I know that I may need to respond to unexpected situations, this birth plan reflects my current intentions. Thank you for helping me have a safe, healthy, and satisfying birth.

n   3. I would like my labor to begin on its own, unless there is a medical reason why induction would be safer.

n   4. I plan to walk, move around, and change positions throughout my labor.

n   5. Other comfort techniques I would like to use:

_____

_____

n   6. I plan to have continuous labor support from a loved one, friend, or doula.

Birth Planning Worksheet *(continued)*

n   7. Names and roles of people I would like to have at my labor:

_____

_____

n   8. I would like my labor room to be quiet and calm.

n   9. Other environment requests:

_____

_____

n   10. I plan to minimize interventions during my labor and birth. I would like to have no routine interventions and intend to avoid the following interventions unless there is a medical reason and assurance that they are safer than the low-tech alternative or doing nothing:

- CONTINUOUS OR INTERMITTENT ELECTRONIC FETAL MONITORING ☐ I prefer intermittent monitoring.
- ARTIFICIAL RUPTURE OF THE MEMBRANES ☐ I would like my waters to break on their own. OR ☐ I am open to the doctor's intervention should that be best for my baby or my own health.
- PITOCIN ☐ I am comfortable with letting labor progress at its own rhythm, and I prefer nondrug methods to help labor progress. OR ☐ I am open to the use of medicine to safely augment labor and delivery at my doctor's approval.

(continued)

From *Cherish the First Six Weeks* © 2013 Helen Moon

Birth Planning Worksheet *(continued)*

- AN INTRAVENOUS LINE ☐ I prefer to eat and drink, but if it is the hospital's policy to start an IV, I would like a saline lock so I can stay mobile.
- EPIDURAL ANALGESIA ☐ I plan to use nondrug methods of pain relief. OR ☐ I am open to the use of an epidural at my doctor's discretion.
- AN EPISIOTOMY ☐ I prefer to let my perineum stretch on its own, and I realize I may experience a natural tear. OR ☐ I would like my doctor to suggest if an episiotomy is necessary.

☐ 11. Other intervention requests:

_____

_____

☐ 12. I don't want to give birth on my back, and I will follow my body's urges to push. OR ☐ I am open to different positions.

☐ 13. Other pushing support I would like to have:

_____

_____

☐ 14. I want to keep my baby with me after birth, allowing us to have as much skin-to-skin contact as possible and unlimited opportunities for breast-feeding. OR ☐ I am open to doctor recommendations for the health and safety of my baby.

THE LOOK OF NEWBORNS

First, not all newborns are so cute and adorable, whether they are born vaginally or by cesarean section. A new baby's head is often too big for her body, she may have skinny chicken legs, and she may look a little battered and bruised, depending on ease of delivery. Newborns may have lots of hair, or no hair, or sparse hair. They may have squinty, swollen, or bloodshot eyes. With a tight delivery, the head can be molded to a point, or be bruised or have a raised bump on the scalp.

A newborn's skin is thin, so the blood vessels can easily be seen below the skin. The baby's skin is often coated with the remains of the vernix, a cheese-like substance that protects the skin in the womb. Some babies have downy prenatal fuzz, usually on their shoulders, back, forehead, and cheeks; this will disappear in the first few weeks. Many babies—both girls and boys—have swollen breasts and/or genitals. This is because of the infusion of female hormones. Some girls may even have vaginal discharge. This is all normal and will go away in the first few weeks.

The Apgar test is given to babies at one minute and five minutes after birth to measure the general condition and assess a newborn at these two critical points. With a score of 7 to 10, the baby is considered in good to excellent condition. A score of 4 to 6 means the baby is in fair condition and may need some assistance. A score of under 4 may require more serious intervention.

Oh, My God! Get This Baby Out—Now!

Feeling huge and tired—and just miserable—is normal when you are about to deliver a baby; actually, these feelings usually signify that you are very close to full term and are ready to give birth.

Here are a few old wives' tales on how to bring on labor and most of the time they work:

1. Go for a walk up a steep hill.
2. Sex! Yes, the same thing that got you here can get you out of it, too! Semen contains a natural prostaglandin that helps the cervix to mature, and orgasm stimulates rhythmic contractions of the uterus.
3. Some pregnancy consultants suggest taking castor oil because it's a natural laxative that can help to bring on labor. However, its effectiveness and safety are arguable. I'd suggest skipping this old wives' recommendation.

The next six chapters offer the details of my CHER-ISH approach to baby care for the first six weeks—one chapter for each week. They focus on how to best feed your child, help him become a regular sleeper, and ease your little one into a schedule that will serve you and your child well in the years to come.

CHAPTER 4

WEEK ONE.
FROM NIGHT TO DAY:
IT'S QUITE A TRANSITION

For any new parent, whether you gave birth to your baby, had a surrogate deliver the baby for you, or are adopting, this week is a giant transition. It is one thing to anticipate and imagine your child and quite another when the baby arrives and is placed in your arms. As exhausted as you may feel from the delivery, or however long it may have been that you were waiting to meet your baby, you now have a little person who is completely dependent on you to keep her warm, fed, and clean, twenty-four hours a day. That's an enormous responsibility—but one that comes with enormous joy.

You have only two goals this week: to take special

care of yourself so that you can recover physically, and to begin to feed, change, and schedule your baby. You both need to get the maximum benefits from the sleep and nutrition that you both need. Your baby is moving from being nocturnal (as he was inside your womb) to becoming used to eating and being awake during the day. Indeed, when you begin to schedule your baby's feedings and sleep, you are helping him learn the difference between night and day. But know this: it isn't an easy transition. You're going to feel waves of physical exhaustion, along with waves of euphoria.

Before you know it, Week One will have passed! So remember to enjoy each moment, as tired and uncomfortable as you may feel.

YOU'RE GOING HOME!

After two or three days in the hospital, most women are ready to go home. Staying in a hospital is exhausting! Constant checks by the nurses, day and night, disrupt your sleep, and depending on your type of delivery, you will be sore and uncomfortable.

Most new moms stay between twenty-four and

forty-eight hours in the hospital, and then are re-leased with their baby. If a baby has been delivered by cesarean, or if a baby or mom is having any kind of health problem, this time frame is extended.

There are a few things you should take home with you from the hospital, like the little pink plastic tub. It can initially be used as a bath, and then used for storing things.

You should definitely keep the blue suction bulb. It really is the only suction bulb that works on those tiny little noses!

Often the hospital will give you extra diapers, wipes, and blankets—feel free to take them home also. The hats and little onesies that your baby uses in the hospital are also yours to keep, as is the bag of mommy items. This mommy bag may include a sitz bottle (a soft squeezy water bottle to help clean your genitals before you can shower); and a sitz bath (a plastic tub that fits onto the top of a toilet seat to clean and soak your bottom and genitals), which will definitely come in handy to help soothe an episiot-omy or hemorrhoids, and also can be used for gen-eral cleaning before you are able to take a shower or bath. The hospital may also give you sanitary nap-kins because, whether you gave birth vaginally or by cesarean, you will bleed for a couple of weeks. The

Some Important Tips for the Hospital

Don't be shy about asking for help
Feed your baby frequently, every two to three hours
Bring home all the little goodies
Painkillers should be used in moderation, as needed

amount of bleeding varies from woman to woman, but you should expect regular bleeding like that which you experience during menstruation.

WHAT'S GOING ON WITH YOUR BABY: WEEK ONE

THE BABY BASICS

• **Sleep** On average, expect your baby to sleep between seventeen and eighteen hours each day. A very sleepy baby does little more than sleep, eat, pee, and poop. Meanwhile, you will be in and out of your own state of euphoria. It's very important, therefore, to wake your baby after three hours so she gets enough

to eat. If she sleeps for too long, she can become le-
thargic and not have the strength to eat enough.

• **Feeding** It is important to feed your baby frequently. Your baby will need to eat every two hours
in the first week. This two- to three-hour period is
from the start of one feed to the start of the next feed.
For example, if you feed your baby at 10:00 A.M.,
you must wake him and feed him again by 1:00 P.M.
A baby's stomach is about the size of a small marble
right now and so it is unable to hold very much milk.
These frequent feedings ensure he gets the nutrition
he needs and also ensures he has enough energy to
keep feeding.

• **Pain medication** Any pain medicine you ingested
during labor and delivery will make your baby sleepier, but it will help you rest and recover a little better.
Try not to take too much, but don't be a martyr and
take too little, either.

• **Birth weight** Your baby can lose up to 10 percent
of his weight in the first few days. This is normal,
so don't worry. If your baby loses any more weight
than that, your pediatrician will recommend the ap-
propriate action. *Always* refer to your pediatrician for
medical advice and begin to keep track of your baby's

weight, week by week, as this is an important measure of the baby's overall health.

• **Baths** During Week One, it is best to simply sponge-bathe your baby, being careful of the genital area if he has been circumcised. It is not necessary or advisable to submerge your baby in water until the umbilical cord falls off.

• **Swaddling** It is important to swaddle your baby after each feeding to help him settle and go back to sleep restfully. Your baby is born with a Moro reflex that causes him to startle frequently. This startle isn't caused by loud noises or bangs; it's simply a reflex and it can awaken him frequently if his arms are free. When he is swaddled, he will feel safe and secure and will sleep better. After all, he is used to a very con-fined space that didn't allow for too much movement.

• **Temperature** Your baby is unable to regulate his temperature right now, so it is important for you to be aware of the temperature of your surroundings. If it is cold, your baby should wear a hat and should stay swaddled in a warm blanket. If it is warm or hot outside, your baby may not need a hat and you should use a lighter blanket. Keep in mind, too, that most heat is lost through the head, so even if it is warm

SWADDLING

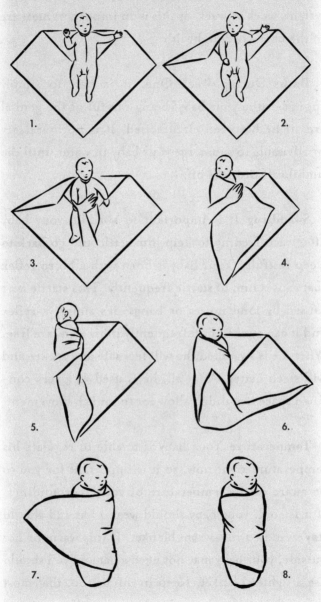

out, check to make sure your baby's body temperature remains warm enough.

YOUR BABY'S REFLEXES

All babies demonstrate instinctive reflexes. Here are some to be aware of:

- **Startle reflex** At sudden loud noises or movements, your baby will startle.

- **Moro reflex** This reflex is when your baby startles involuntarily (not to be confused with the startle reflex).

- **Rooting reflex** If you stroke your baby's cheek gently, she will turn in the direction of the stimulus, open her mouth, and be ready to suckle.

- **Walking or stepping reflex** When held upright on a hard, flat surface, a newborn will lift his legs and take "steps."

- **Palmar grasp** Place your finger in the baby's palm, and it will cause a flexing of her hand and she will grasp your finger. A newborn's grasp is powerful enough to support her full body weight.

• **Babinski reflex** If the sole of your baby's foot is gently stroked from heel to toe, the toes will flare upward and the foot will turn in.

CIRCUMCISION

Remember, this procedure is often harder for the parents than it is for the baby. He will have forgotten all about it as soon as it is finished.

To care for the area afterward, apply petroleum jelly at each diaper change. I usually use gauze pads, put the petroleum jelly on the pad, and then cover the tip of the penis with it. You can be quite generous with the jelly, as we don't want anything sticking to the penis. Make sure that the petroleum jelly is pure, without perfumes or other additives.

If your doctor sent you home with an antibiotic ointment, you will want to use this as directed. Quite often, the head of the penis will have a dressing wrapped around it; be sure not to pull it off unless you are supposed to. Follow the instructions from your doctor or *mohel*. Do not bathe your son for at least the first week, but do wash the penis frequently.

Contact your doctor or *mohel* immediately if there is any:

Swelling
Bleeding (other than just a drop or two)

Foul-smelling discharge

Difficulty urinating

Fever

Black or blue discoloration

Consistent redness that appears suddenly and
    does not disappear after a few days

BIRTHMARKS

Birthmarks can be flat or raised, have regular or ir-
regular borders, and be different shades of color
ranging from brown, tan, black, and pale blue to
pink, red, or purple. The two main types of birthmarks are red, which are vascular birthmarks (for example, "strawberry" hemangiomas, port-wine stains,
and "stork bites"), and pigmented birthmarks (such
as moles, café-au-lait spots, and Mongolian spots).

The types of birthmarks are differentiated by their
causes. Vascular (blood vessel) birthmarks happen
when blood vessels don't form correctly; either there
are too many of them or they're wider than usual
and get tangled together. Pigmented birthmarks are
caused by an overgrowth of the cells that create pigment in skin. Most birthmarks are benign and many
even go away on their own or shrink over time. A doctor should evaluate a birthmark when it first appears
to determine its type and what kind of monitoring
and treatment it needs, if any. Sometimes birthmarks

are associated with other health problems, so talk to your doctor about whether this might be the case for your child. Call the doctor if a birthmark ever bleeds, hurts, itches, or becomes infected. Birthmarks can't be prevented, and they're not caused by anything done or not done during pregnancy. There's no truth to old wives' tales about "stains" being caused by something the mother did or ate. The cause of most birthmarks is unknown. They can be inherited, but usually are not, and typically are unrelated to trauma to the skin during childbirth.

JAUNDICE

Babies become jaundiced when they have too much bilirubin in their blood. Bilirubin is a normal pigment made when red blood cells break down in the body. It is usually processed by the liver, recycled, and eliminated in the baby's stool. When a baby has jaundice, it means either that his body is making too much bilirubin or the liver is not getting rid of it quickly enough.

Feeding (especially breast-feeding) your baby often in the first hours and days after birth helps reduce the risk of jaundice. Your baby will pass more stool, and the milk will give your baby's liver the energy it needs to process the bilirubin. Most jaundice is not harmful to your baby. It usually shows up during the baby's first three to five days of life, then disappears as the baby's body learns to deal with bilirubin.

If the level of bilirubin becomes very high, it may affect some of the baby's brain cells. This may cause the baby to be less active. In rare cases, a baby may develop seizures (convulsions). The effects of this kind of jaundice may also lead to deafness, cerebral palsy, and/or serious developmental delay. Fortunately, it can usually be prevented. One way to reduce bilirubin levels is to expose the baby's skin to light, a process called phototherapy. The baby's eyes are protected from the light by eye patches. With phototherapy, the baby may have skin rashes or loose bowel movements. He may need to take in extra fluids (such as via more frequent breast-feeding). Phototherapy is safe, but it is only used when needed (usually for two to three days). In severe cases, the baby may need to be given fluids intravenously or through a blood transfusion.

STOOL COLOR

In the first couple of days, your baby will pass meconium, a sticky green-black substance made up of bile, mucus, and amniotic fluid that builds up in her system while she is in the womb. Babies usually start passing meconium twelve hours after birth; this is a sign that the bowel system is healthy and functioning properly.

If your baby doesn't pass meconium within the first twenty-four hours, it could be a sign of intestinal obstruction, and you should contact your physician. Once the meconium is expelled from the body, expect your baby's poop to change in color to brown-green and in texture from loose and grainy to increasingly yellow with the consistency of grainy mustard.

Sneezing, Hiccups, and Shivering

It is completely normal for your baby to sneeze a lot, get the hiccups, and quiver a little. Babies sneeze frequently because their nasal passageways are so tiny that the slightest tickle can irritate their noses. Hiccups are caused by sudden contractions of the diaphragm as a result of irritation or stimulation of that muscle. These hiccups are usually caused by feeding or a drop in temperature that causes a baby to get cold.

Babies with gastro-esophageal reflux disease may hiccup more frequently. Hiccups do not harm your child or cause her pain. And there's really not much you can do; they'll go away soon.

You may notice your baby's lip quiver from time

to time or her little body shiver occasionally. This is all normal—the body shivering is a reflex and the lip quivering is just the sign of an immature nervous system.

BREAST-FEEDING

The prospect of breast-feeding can seem a little daunting when you are doing it the first time. The best thing you can do is to relax. Your baby has strong instincts to nurse, and you just need to guide him a little.

You always need to support your breast with your free hand when offering it to your baby. I have seen a few moms try to push their babies to the breast and expect the babies to know how nurse; sadly, this isn't so. Remember, you have to teach your baby how to do *everything*: he has just come from a perfect little environment where everything was easy and he just had to hang out and enjoy; now he has to do a little more work.

Don't be shy about asking for help with breast-feeding. Most hospitals have a lactation consultant available, so take advantage of the hands-on professional demonstration or advice. And don't hesitate to ask the lactation consultant to slow down and answer your questions. At busy hospitals and birthing centers, these consultants can become very harried, but it is their job to advise you on how to make breast-feeding become a little easier.

GETTING STARTED WITH FEEDING

If you've decided that you want to give breast-feeding a try, here are some basics:

1. **START EARLY.** Let your Ob-Gyn know you're going to nurse so you can feed your baby straight after delivery. It can take up to an hour after birth for the baby to want to latch on, but this is the best start you and your baby can have.

2. **STAY TOGETHER.** As mentioned earlier, breast-feeding is hindered when your baby is away in the hospital nursery. If you can't see when your baby is hungry, how do you know when your baby is ready to eat? For this reason, I encourage you to request that your baby be near you while you two are still in the hospital.

3. **PRACTICE.** In the first couple of days, your baby does not need a large volume of milk, but she does need to nurse. This is a time not to worry about amounts, but to concentrate on technique. The small

amounts of colostrum you are producing are more than sufficient for your baby, and her stomach can't tolerate much more.

4. **FEED ON DEMAND.** In those first few days, feed the baby when she's hungry; that's always best for the baby and your milk supply. However, do not let the baby sleep more than three and a half hours, or she can become too weak to eat.

5. **NO BOTTLES NEEDED.** Do not allow the nursing staff to give your baby a bottle of formula or sugar water, as this will curb your baby's appetite and hinder nursing. Unless your baby has some medical need, she does not need extra fluids!

6. **PATIENCE IS NECESSARY.** Remember, neither you nor your baby has done this before; you both have to learn. So be patient and remember that if your labor was long and difficult, your baby is probably tired also.

7. **STAY CALM.** No matter how difficult it gets, tension can affect your letdown (your letdown is when your milk starts to flow), so it is absolutely necessary to stay as relaxed as possible. Make yourself comfortable; don't allow visitors when nursing. Take deep breaths before beginning a breast-feeding—read a book, watch TV, or whatever else will relax you before you begin.

LATCHING ON

Your baby will learn to latch on, but please know it may take a few attempts for the two of you to work out your system. Since all women's nipples are shaped differently, it's important that you find the best position and best way to bring your baby to your breast.

The illustrations below demonstrate how to help your baby latch.

LATCHING ON

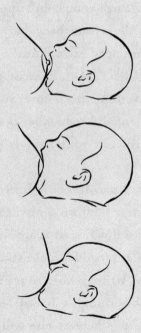

Here is a general guide for achieving the best results:

1. Tickle you baby's lips with your nipple until her mouth opens really wide, like a yawn.

2. When your baby's mouth is wide open, pull her close to take as much of your areola in her mouth as possible, so her jaws don't close on your nipple. By positioning the baby's mouth back from the nipple, her suckling will stimulate the milk ducts to bring the milk forward into the nipple area. This will ensure your baby gets as much milk as possible and will help prevent nipple soreness.

3. When well-positioned at the breast, the baby's lips will be flanged out and her tongue cupped at the bottom of your nipple, with her chin touching the lower part of your breast. This is what is referred to as "latching on."

4. Your baby should breathe easily, with nostrils flared. If she seems to have trouble breathing, lift your breast a little or pull her legs a little closer to you so her nose pulls away slightly from the breast. Don't push on your breast to move it away from her nose because this action may pull your nipple out of the back of her mouth, which could cause soreness to your nipple.

5. Let your baby breast-feed until she lets go of the breast, but try and keep an eye on the time that has passed. (At the end of this chapter, you will find a sample log for tracking your baby's sleep and feeding schedule as well as room to write down comments.) You might try burping your baby, although some breast-fed babies don't burp very much, especially between breasts.

6. Switch breasts.

7. Be careful when removing your baby from your breast. If her gums rub across your nipples, it will hurt and your nipples may become sore. I suggest gently putting your finger between her gums to break the suction and holding your finger there to protect your nipple while removing your nipple and breast from the baby's mouth.

Continue to offer both breasts at each nursing session because it will help establish your milk supply. Start the next nursing on the last breast offered or, if for some reason your baby only nursed on one side, offer the breast that your baby didn't take at the last feeding. It's easy to remember which breast to offer first because that side will feel fuller. Remember that it is normal for one breast to make more milk than the other and for your baby to prefer one breast to the other.

At first you may feel a stretching sensation as your baby starts to pull your nipple into her mouth. For some women the feeling may be slightly painful, but it goes away quickly during feeding and fades after a few days. If your baby tends to arch backward and pull away, tucking her legs in on the other side of your body will help keep her attached and breast-feeding effectively.

During the first week after delivery, oftentimes on the third or fourth day, your milk supply will increase. That's when moms say that their milk has "come in," which is not exactly accurate, as your body has produced milk from the time your baby was born. Gradually your milk will change from colostrum to transitional to mature milk during the next few weeks. *Colostrum* is early milk produced during pregnancy and readily available the first thirty-six to seventy-two hours after birth. *Transitional milk* is a mix of colostrum and mature milk produced between days three and fourteen. *Mature milk* develops about two weeks after giving birth and appears thinner than cow's milk. It may look slightly blue, although the color varies from woman to woman, and it may be affected by diet.

As long as you breast-feed, your milk will change to meet your baby's needs. For instance, at the beginning of a nursing session, your milk is plentiful and high in carbohydrates. Toward the end of the nursing session, you produce *hind-milk*, a creamy milk that is high in fat and calories and is very filling for your baby.

If you want to pump your milk to store extra, don't start until at least the second week after your baby is born. By pumping too early, you may end up making more milk than you need, or getting too engorged. You would need to pump sooner only if your milk supply were poor and you were trying to stimulate production, or if your baby was unable to nurse for medical reasons and you wanted your baby to still have breast milk. In any of these cases, it's best to seek advice from a lactation consultant or pediatrician before beginning to pump and store in Week Two.

KEEP A LOG

Moms find it very difficult to keep track of the feeding schedule during Week One, which is why I advise keeping a log of when your baby feeds and also when he pees and poops. This is the best way for you to know that your baby is getting enough milk. The hospital usually provides a chart for you, or you can use the one provided at the end of this chapter (see page 124). Keeping track of this information will also help your baby's doctor, especially if any health problems arise.

Before leaving the hospital, it is especially important to know how frequently your baby is peeing. If
your baby has jaundice, for instance, the frequency
of pee will help let the doctors know whether the bilirubin is passing through the baby's body or accumu-
lating in higher levels.

Remember, babies suck reflexively; the sucking
does not always suggest that your baby is still hungry.
Reflexive suckling means that baby will suck on anything that is put in or near his mouth. In fact, a baby
may empty a bottle of water or formula, right after
breast-feeding, owing to this reflex.

IF YOU NEED TO OR DECIDE TO STOP

One mom I worked with had nursed her baby for a
week, and then she became ill with a fever and infection. To help reduce and then stop her milk supply,
she pumped a little less time each morning and then
used one of nature's little miracles: green cabbage
leaves. Green cabbage has a chemical in it that helps
to dry up your milk.

If you place a cold cabbage leaf on each breast
under your bra and leave them there for an hour or
two each day, it will lessen your supply (if you would
like to decrease the amount), but don't leave them on
too long if you want to continue to breast-feed; this is
very effective and you don't want to hinder the supply

that you need for your baby. However, if for whatever reason you wish to stop nursing, cabbage leaves will dry up your milk altogether.

FORMULA AND BOTTLES

• • • • • •

If you have decided to bottle-feed your baby, the hospital will provide prefilled disposable bottles and nipples. This formula from the hospital is absolutely fine to use unless your family has a history of lactose, dairy, or soy intolerances. In that case, you should discuss the formula options beforehand with your doctor, so that you can be prepared. However, most milk intolerances don't show up until the second week, after you have brought your baby home.

Either way, if you know of a family history of dietary intolerances, it's best to be prepared with a couple of different types of formula. Even though some women find bottle-feeding to be easier than breast-feeding, preparing the formula and sterilizing the bottles takes a lot more time and work.

Choosing a Formula

In general, you want a formula that is as close to breast milk as possible. Similac, Enfamil, and Gerber Good Start are the most common. Organic formulas are also available, as are alternatives for babies with food allergies and metabolic disorders. You will find formula in ready-to-use bottles, ready-to-pour cans, and ready-to-mix powders. You will have to weigh the benefits of convenience versus cost when you choose.

Preparing the Bottles

Always wash your hands before preparing the bottles and wash everything to be used for feeding your baby with hot, soapy water, then rinse thoroughly.

Check the expiration dates on cans of ready-to-pour formula; do not use formula after the use-by date has expired.

Wash the top of the can with hot, soapy water before opening it. Use a sharp, clean can opener, and keep it for this use only.

If using powdered formula, follow the directions on the can. Level off the scoops of powder and do not pack them down.

If you use room-temperature water, you don't have to warm the bottle, but if the formula has been refrigerated, then it must be warmed. To test that the formula is the right temperature, tip a drop on to the back of your wrist. It should feel neither cold nor hot.

VISITORS AT HOME

Once you are home from the hospital, everyone under the sun will want to pop by and see your new baby. But it is important to limit the visitors, for a number of reasons. First, the more people who visit, the more you are exposing your new baby to germs during a time when his immune system is in overdrive, building up its stamina and its strength. All visitors should wash their hands as they enter your house, and especially before touching the baby. Don't be shy about asking them to do this.

Second, if you are entertaining guests, you are wasting precious time when you could be resting. Remember, the guests happily go home and sleep all night; you, on the other hand, are going to be up every two to three hours feeding and caring for your baby. So limit your guests initially to family only, and if you have a big family, ask them not to stay too long.

Your baby is also transitioning into the world, and it's better for him to have a calm, relaxed environment in which to adjust. Overstimulation can lead to your baby's becoming unnecessarily fussy and not able to get the sleep he needs. A tired and fussy baby also has trouble eating, leading to poor weight gain and less milk production for you—it can be a vicious cycle that is hard to break.

The same can be true for you. When a new mom doesn't get the rest she needs, she will produce less milk. You should try to get a minimum of eight hours of sleep a day. A good rule of thumb is this: for every three hours you are awake during the night, you will need to sleep an extra two hours during the day. Broken sleep (during the night) is not as restful and replenishing as unbroken sleep. By including a two-hour nap during the day, you give your body and brain the extra sleep necessary to stay healthy. Indeed, some experts are now researching the link between exhaustion and postpartum depression, and the likelihood that exhaustion triggers or exacerbates the postpartum blues.

Many new moms feel guilty about asking for the time to nap. One mom with whom I worked worried about taking away adult time from her husband, who had a job that kept him out late at night. Mom felt she needed to stay up until he came home so that they could spend some time together. But she was exhausted by that late in the day!

So I suggested a compromise: she would go to bed

early, when she was tired, and if she heard her husband come home, then she could get up and spend time with him. If she woke up to spend time with her husband, then she had to take a good nap during the day. The result? The woman often slept through her husband's return home and began to feel physically stronger and more emotionally balanced. Her husband, of course, didn't mind at all—he was relieved that his wife was feeling better.

START THE SCHEDULE RIGHT AWAY

A s soon as you are home and comfortable, start a feeding and sleeping schedule. This means that you feed your baby every two and a half to three hours every day and night in the first week. If your baby is still asleep after three hours at nighttime only, you may let him sleep a little longer, but no more than four hours. This typically doesn't happen in the first week because your baby is getting small amounts of milk and will be hungry. However, if you are bottle-feeding, you can happily let your baby sleep up to four or five hours, although again this is unlikely in the first week.

As you might guess, this schedule will not be easy on you or your partner. To make matters a bit more challenging, it's very common for babies to be fussy at any time during the night, but especially during the witching hour, between 5:00 and 7:00 P.M. That is, babies tend to appear hungry even when they are not. Try to hold off! It will be difficult in the beginning, but it will pay off quickly.

After a couple of fussy nights when you feel exhausted and the baby is acting like she needs to be fed every hour, she will begin to adjust: she will be less nocturnal and more used to sleeping at night. Of course, she will still sleep a lot during the day as well, with several little awake periods.

Remember, it's natural and healthy for your baby to sleep between fifteen and eighteen hours in a twenty-four-hour period. She will most likely eat eight times in that same time period, and will be awake eating about half an hour to an hour; that doesn't leave very much time for your baby to be awake. Don't try to keep her awake to get her to sleep longer. IT DOESN'T WORK THAT WAY! The old saying with babies is, "Sleep begets sleep." So the better rested your baby is, the better she will sleep.

Be Careful of a Snacking Baby!

Babies get sleepy very quickly, so you need to encourage your baby to eat and not just snack! If the feed is too short and she snacks, then you will have a fussy, hungry baby very quickly. By encouraging your baby to feed for fifteen to twenty minutes on each side, you will feel more confident in knowing she ate sufficiently so that if she wakes a little early, you know she's okay to wait!

The Love Hormone

The hormone oxytocin is often called the "love" or "happy" hormone. The oxytocin your body produces after giving birth has a number of roles, two of which are the following:

1. It helps trigger the milk letdown after the colostrum comes. When your baby first sucks on your nipples, that sends a signal to your brain that releases the oxytocin, thereby also releasing the milk in your breasts.
2. It helps you bond with your baby. After delivery, there is an increased concentration of oxytocin levels in the brain. Scientific studies have shown how this hormone makes the mother more nurturing, patient, and protective of her baby.

Gentle Tactics for Waking a Sleeping Baby

- Undress the baby
- Give gentle tickles
- Rub your finger under the baby's chin to encourage sucking
- Play with the baby's feet
- Run your finger gently down your baby's back
- Change your baby's diaper
- If all else fails, get a cool, wet washcloth and wipe baby's face, hands, and back

WEEK ONE SCHEDULE

Your daily schedule with your baby at home is going to look a little like this if you are breast-feeding:

SCHEDULE FOR BREAST-FED BABIES _____

7:00 A.M.	Unswaddle the baby and change his diaper; feed 15 to 20 minutes on each side; burp well in between breasts and after
9:30 A.M.	Feeding
12 noon	Feeding
2:30 P.M.	Feeding

5:00 P.M.   Feeding

7:30 P.M.   Feeding

10:00 P.M.   Feeding

1:00 A.M.   Feeding

4:00 A.M.   Feeding

7:00 A.M.   Feeding (starting the next day's
              schedule)

This is a very typical first-week schedule. The main goal is to make sure the night feeds are every three hours. I make sure that every night the baby is fed at 10:00 P.M., no matter what time the last feeding was. It may have been less than two and a half hours, but I still feed the baby at 10:00 P.M. This is the only time of day that you should break the two-and-a-half- to three-hour feeding rule.

Ultimately your baby will get used to this feeding at 10:00 P.M. and it will be the start of his long night sleep. So, if you fed your baby at 8:00 P.M., then feed him again at 10:00 P.M., no matter what. Or, if he is due to eat at 9:00 P.M., then feed him sooner so you can squeeze in another feeding at 10:00 P.M. Try to work the feedings so you have at least two hours between the last feeding and the 10:00 P.M. feeding.

The more consistent you can be with the 10:00 P.M. feeding, the sooner your baby will get into the habit of this being his last feeding for the night. It is so tempting during the night to want to feed your baby sooner if he wakes up and is fussy, but try not to; he may settle down if you reswaddle him, reposition him, or give him a few little pats and some shushing. Only feed him if all else fails.

Someone once said to me, "You don't need to burp a breast-fed baby, right?" Wrong. It is just as important to burp breast-fed babies as it is bottle-fed babies; they just don't burp as loudly or as frequently. A bottle-fed baby's burps tend to come up loud and quickly; a breast-fed baby's burps are much quieter in general, and easier to miss. Occasionally you won't get a burp, but you should still try for it. It all comes down to how much air your baby takes in when she eats; her latch on your breast will be much tighter and so she takes in less air, making her burps less strong. But if you have a baby who is pulling on and off the breast frequently, chances are he will take in more air and will need more burping.

There is nothing worse than getting your baby relaxed and settled down to sleep, only to be woken up twenty minutes later because she is uncomfortable and needs to burp or has spit up everywhere, because the burp came up with some of the milk she was drinking. You may need to change your baby's diaper again after the feeding, and sometimes during the feeding, as she will have frequent poops when breast-feeding. Most pediatricians will tell you it is normal for your baby to poop once a day or ten times a day.

After the feeding and burping, swaddle your baby and hold him for a little while for the food to digest. During the day, when you have just finished feeding and burping your baby, this is a great time to interact with him. You can talk to him or sing to him, looking into his eyes, rubbing his head—babies love this. It's very relaxing and comforting to him. Once he is getting sleepy, then gently place your baby in his bassinet or crib.

A bottle-fed baby's daily schedule in the first week will look a little like this:

SCHEDULE FOR BOTTLE-FED BABIES_____
7:00 A.M.   Bottle-feed
10:00 A.M.   Bottle-feed
1:00 P.M.   Bottle-feed
4:00 P.M.   Bottle-feed
7:00 P.M.   Bottle-feed
10:00 P.M.   Bottle-feed
1:00 A.M.   Bottle-feed
4:00 A.M.   Bottle-feed

7:00 A.M.   Bottle-feed (starting the next day's schedule)

Again, you will change your baby before the feeding, and after if necessary, and burp throughout the feeding. A bottle-fed baby's burps come up loud and quickly; you can actually feel the burp move through his little body. He will often have a couple of burps, so don't stop on the first burp.

If you are bottle-feeding, it is a little easier to keep your baby on a three-hour schedule, as she will feel fuller for longer with the formula. The most important point to remember when feeding formula with a bottle is that you must get the burps up after each feeding.

Generally in the first week your baby will probably eat about 1 ounce to a maximum of 2 ounces at a feeding. So I recommend burping your baby after each half ounce. If you have a particularly hungry baby, then let her have up to an ounce and then burp her, but make sure you get a good burp or two before you offer any more milk. In the first week, your baby will poop frequently when bottle-feeding.

TECHNIQUES FOR BURPING

t is important to hold your baby correctly to make burping easier. In the first three weeks, it is easier to burp your baby when she is seated on your lap, with one hand supporting her head at the front and your other hand rubbing her back in a firm, rhythmic, upward motion. (See the illustrations on the facing page for how to place your hands.)

Alternatively, place your baby on your shoulder with his head resting on top of your shoulder and again firmly rub his back in an upward rhythmic motion. I have found that many parents tend not to pat their baby as firmly as they need to in order to release the burps. A soft, gentle pat will have very little to no effect at all.

If you are still finding it difficult to encourage your baby to release a burp, then try this little trick: gently and slowly lay your baby across your knees so he is flat, and then just as gently bring him upright again. This gentle motion will often help move the position of the trapped air and allow the burp to come up more easily. If you keep your baby in the same position the whole time you are burping, the trapped air will often tend to sit there. If this still doesn't work, then another little trick is to lay your

BURPING TECHNIQUES

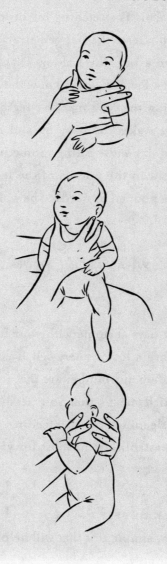

baby face down across your knees and gently rub his back from his bottom to his head in the same rhythmic motion. This is stretching his little tummy and again can help release the trapped air.

I am often asked why I always change the baby's diaper before a feeding, as we know the baby will pee or poop during the feeding. The reason is that the diaper change wakes the baby up and allows her to feel clean and dry while eating. Sometimes you have to change again in the middle of the feeding, as the baby may have pooped or needs to be woken up again.

WHAT ABOUT *YOU?*

In those first days at home with your baby, you may appear to have a lot of energy. It is coming mostly from the excitement, but beware that the energy will fade fast, which means that you need to rest when the baby is sleeping. So the feeding and sleeping schedule you establish is not just for your baby; it is also for you.

BREAST MILK SUPPLY

Here are a few simple tips that will help you establish a good milk supply:

- **Liquids.** You need to drink a lot. You will find you are thirstier than you have ever been before. You should try to drink a glass of water before, during, or after every feed.

- **Food.** Eat when you are hungry and try not to skip meals. If you are having visitors and they ask if they can bring anything for you, ask for food. There is nothing better than having prepared meals and healthful snacks you can grab when needed.

- **Stimulation of the breasts.** The most effective stimulation is having your baby nurse consistently. He should nurse at least fifteen to twenty minutes on both sides; so if your baby falls asleep, wake him up!

ENGORGEMENT

When a new mom's breast milk comes in, her breasts will feel very heavy, uncomfortable, and actually painful. This is called *engorgement* and it's not only normal, it means everything is working the way it should. The best way to relieve breast engorgement is to feed your baby. However, because your breasts are so full, a simple feeding may not be enough to relieve the fullness. In fact, some babies may even appear to be choking on the sudden volume of milk that you are producing.

So how do you deal with this? First, you need to take care of the discomfort you are feeling. I always recommend a warm compresses before feeding. The best way to make a compress is to use a disposable diaper, run the hot water and get the inside of the diaper wet. Make sure the water is not scalding—you don't want to burn yourself. Then place the diaper over your breasts; you can actually use the tabs so that the diaper cups your breasts, or just put your bra over the diaper to hold it in place. Do this fifteen minutes before each feed; it will feel so good! It also helps with the letdown. Then, if you are still in some discomfort after the feeding, use a cold compress. You could also hold a bag of frozen peas against the skin of your breasts (across the nipples) for up to thirty minutes.

The worst thing to do for engorgement is to pump! Because breast milk works on a supply-and-demand process, the more you demand, whether by nursing or pumping, the more the breasts will produce. By pumping, you are asking for more milk than your baby needs.

The only exception to this rule is when you have such an abundance of milk that your baby begins to choke because of the copious flow. Then, I recommend pumping for two to three minutes *before* each feeding to help avoid the initial flood of milk.

Typically, engorgement lasts for about four or five days, after which point you should start to feel less swollen and uncomfortable. You should be able to stop the pumping before each feeding at this point, if that's what you have had to do.

C-SECTION RECOVERY

What other comfort or health problems might you face in your first week? This depends a lot on your type of delivery. If you delivered by cesarean, you are going to be more uncomfortable than if you had a vaginal birth. A c-section is the equivalent of having major abdominal surgery. When you have major abdominal surgery, you need rest to recuperate. When you have a baby, though, you don't get a whole lot of time to do that.

Having your baby, however, is going to help make the recovery from a c-section easier and quicker. Part of this is due to your hormones. There is a higher abundance of oxytocin, or as some refer to it, the happy/love hormone. When your baby suckles at your breasts, oxytocin is released and you feel happy. This will help in your recovery.

But expect a lot of discomfort. It will be difficult to sit up and move around too quickly. Laughing will hurt. It will be difficult to get up and go to the bathroom, so you will probably have a catheter for the first day or two in the hospital. I have seen some moms get out of bed the next day and be mobile relatively easily, but others have a harder time.

After a cesarean, it is important to get up and move about, but it is just as important to make sure you don't overdo it. Watch out for infections in the incision, although this doesn't typically happen in the first week. The most important challenge is keeping your incision clean. Though you don't want to shower too frequently, it is important to gently wash the incision area and pat it as dry as possible.

VAGINAL BIRTH RECOVERY

After a vaginal birth, women have varying degrees of discomfort. If you were lucky enough to have a delivery that was smooth, quick, and with no tearing, then your discomfort will be minimal. If you had an episiotomy or a tear occurred during the birth, you have probably had stitches; this can be pretty painful. Your doctor will suggest you get out of bed to sit in a chair or walk.

The top part of your uterus is called the fundus. After vaginal delivery, your uterus will start to return to its normal size and your fundus will get harder. This helps control the bleeding. Your fundus will be checked often during the first hour after delivery, and as needed thereafter. Your doctor may push gently on your abdomen to feel how soft or hard your fundus is.

As your body returns to postpartum state, you will bleed. You may pass a blood clot; any clot smaller than 2 inches is normal. If you pass a clot that is larger than 2 inches, contact your physician. The same is true of the bleeding as your tissue restores itself. If you are filling more than one or two pads every one or two hours, you should contact your physician. Activity will help your circulation and can help prevent blood clots from forming.

Here are a few things you should do to care for yourself after a vaginal delivery:

• **Constipation and hemorrhoids.** You may have constipation and hemorrhoids for a period of time after you have your baby. Constipation is defined as hard bowel movements that are difficult to pass. Hemorrhoids are swollen veins around or in your rectum that may cause you pain. Ask your doctor what you should do about preventing constipation and how to care for the hemorrhoids.

• **Perineal care.** Keep your perineum (the soft tissue between your anus and vagina) clean to help prevent an infection. Your doctor will probably suggest using sitz baths. You can use warm- or cold-water sitz baths, but cold baths may help relieve pain more quickly. Your doctor should give you more information about how to take sitz baths. If you have stitches in your perineum, wash the area gently with soap and water when you bathe or shower.

• **Vaginal discharge.** You will have vaginal discharge, called lochia, after your delivery. The lochia is bright red the first day or two after the birth. By the third or fourth day, the amount decreases, and it turns a pinkish color. Sometimes the discharge has a slight odor. You may need to wear a pad and change it many times each day. It is normal to have lochia up to eight weeks after your baby is born.

If you had an episiotomy during your vaginal birth, you may want to sit on a Boppy cushion or a neck pillow to relieve some of the pressure on the vaginal area. This can make it a lot more comfortable when you are breast feeding, too. You can also use a bag of ice to help ease some of the pain when you are not feeding.

Night Sweats

Toward the end of the first week, you may experience night sweats. This is also normal; it is merely your body releasing the excess fluids that have built up in the end of your pregnancy and during delivery. The sweating can be profuse, even to the point where you may need to change your clothes in the middle of the night! I have known moms who have thrown away their pillows because the amount of sweat during this period has made the pillow smell so bad. Thankfully, the sweating usually doesn't last for more than two weeks. But do expect to feel warmer than usual, simply because of the extra work your body is doing to produce the milk and regulate your hormones.

Your baby is brand-new to the world, but he already knows some things about you. He will be familiar with your smell and your voice. Any time you feed, hold, change, or talk to your baby, you are helping him settle into the brand-new world around him. All of these interactions help to foster your bond, soothe your baby, and begin that life-long relationship based on safety, trust, and love.

Just as your baby makes his way through this transition week, you are helping him get ready for the next chapter: In Week Two, you will see how even after just seven days, your baby will begin to change!

Baby·Chart

DATE	TIME	BREAST-FEEDING (minutes/breast)		FORMULA-FEEDING (in ounces)	DIAPER CHANGES		ASLEEP/ AWAKE	COMMENTS
		Left	Right		Wet (W)	Poop (P)		
	7:00 A.M.							
	9:45 A.M.							
	12:45 P.M.							
	3:30 P.M.							
	6:15 P.M.							
	9:00 P.M.							
	12:00 A.M.							
	2:30 A.M.							
	5:30 A.M.							
	8:15 A.M.							

From *Cherish the First Six Weeks* © 2013 Helen Moon

DATE	TIME	BREAST-FEEDING (minutes/breast)		FORMULA-FEEDING (in ounces)	DIAPER CHANGES		ASLEEP/ AWAKE	COMMENTS
		Left	Right		Wet (W)	Poop (P)		
1/1/10	7:00 A.M.	15 min.	15 min.		W	P x 2	asleep @ 7:45 am awake @ 9:35 am	a little fussy
	9:45 A.M.	15 min.	20 min.		W	P	asleep @ 10:45 am awake @ 12:35 pm	wouldn't settle
	12:45 P.M.	15 min.	15 min. ✔		W	P	asleep @ 2:00 pm	good feed
	3:30 P.M.							
	6:15 P.M.							
	9:00 P.M.							
	12:00 A.M.							
	2:30 A.M.							
	5:30 A.M.							
	8:15 A.M.							

✔ Last breast offered

From *Cherish the First Six Weeks* © 2013 Helen Moon

CHAPTER 5

WEEK TWO.
ENJOY: IT'S YOUR
HONEYMOON!

I call Week Two the Honeymoon Stage. Why? Because as long as your baby is eating well—your milk flow is well established if you are nursing, and she doesn't have any problems with formula if you are bottle-feeding—then you should find that your baby does little more than eat, sleep, pee, and poop. Perhaps you're feeling quite over the top with exhaustion, though, and wondering how I might ever call this the honeymoon. Perhaps you even find the term misleading if you are still up, feeding your baby every three hours, day and night.

Most babies are still sleeping around fifteen to

eighteen hours a day. Even though your baby is pretty sleepy after every feeding, there should definitely be more of a rhythm to the feeding schedule and less fussiness between feedings during the night. You may still be on a pain medication if you had a c-section, a bad tear, or another painful condition and this will contribute to your baby's sleepy state also.

Your baby could also be sleepy during his feedings and so will need encouragement to eat sufficiently. (Remember the tactics for waking a sleeping baby: undress the baby, gently tickle, rub your finger under the baby's chin to encourage sucking, play with the baby's feet, run your finger gently down the baby's back. If all else fails, get a cool, wet washcloth and wipe the baby's face, hands, and back.)

By now your baby should be quite happy to be swaddled and settled down to sleep at nighttime, either in a bassinet, co-sleeper (a type of bassinet that hooks onto the side of your bed), or crib. I don't recommend having your baby sleep with you in your bed. First, you won't sleep so well yourself, missing out on that little valuable sleep you get. The moms who I have seen sleep with their babies have all told me the same thing—they constantly wake up at every little twitch or noise their baby makes. Believe me, you will still hear your baby if she is in her own bed.

The second reason I don't recommend sleeping with your baby is that your baby will become dependent on your warm body being there beside her.

I worked weekends for a family that had three children. When I arrived, the kids were all sleeping with their parents. The ages of the kids? Seven, five, and two—that's years, not months! Why was I there, you may be wondering? So that the parents could go away for the weekend in their RV to have some private time together.

However, using the same basic method that I use with newborn babies, I helped settle the children in their respective rooms, and on the very first night all three children slept in their own beds and continued to do so each night that I was there, as well as after their parents returned home. Isn't it better to have your private time every night and to teach your baby to happily sleep in her own space?

If you feel more comfortable having your baby's bassinet or crib in your room in the first few months, I am all for that; it also makes it easier to get up and down each night to feed the baby. You may want to have a little changing station in your room, also.

This is also often the time when a new mom feels compelled to check on her baby's breathing. There is so much information out there about sudden infant death syndrome (SIDS) that it makes us all worry.

When a baby is sleeping so hard and soundly, it's only natural to want to check on him. I find myself doing it with certain babies, even after all my years of experience. I don't think it's a bad thing to do—it just shows that you care—but just do so without disturbing your sleeping baby. Whenever you have the need to check on your baby, first look to see if his chest is moving up and down. You could also put your hand in front of his mouth to feel his breath.

WEEK TWO SCHEDULE

● ● ● ● ● ●

The baby's schedule is going to be very similar to that of the first week: you will feed your baby every two and a half to three hours, depending on whether you are nursing or bottle-feeding formula. If you are nursing, the two-and-a-half-hour period during the day stimulates a good supply of breast milk and your baby gets enough nutrition during this critical time.

These first two weeks play a pivotal role in your milk production. Each time you nurse, your body knows that it needs to make more milk. So even if your baby is sleeping, you should try to stick to the schedule and gently rouse your baby to eat. If you have a particularly sleepy baby, then it is going to feel like you are constantly waking your baby for a feeding, but this is necessary for your milk production. Sometimes this will mean that your baby is eating later than the two-and-a-half-hour mark, as it may have taken you fifteen or twenty minutes to wake your baby up sufficiently to eat. This can happen frequently, but what you may see happening is that you have to wake your baby for one feeding, then she will wake herself for the next, thereby keeping her on the two-and-a-half- to three-hour cycle.

You also want to ensure your baby is eating sufficiently, so that when she goes to the doctor for her two-week checkup and weigh-in, she has gained her birth weight back, as this will then allow you to start stretching her nighttime feedings and allowing my recommended sleep routine to begin!

SCHEDULE FOR BREAST-FED BABIES _____

7:00 A.M.   Unswaddle the baby and change
              his diaper; nurse, 15 to 20 minutes
              on each side; burp well in between
              breasts and after
9:30 A.M.   Feeding
12 noon   Feeding
2:30 P.M.   Feeding
5:00 P.M.   Feeding

Gentle Reminder of Flow of Feeding

Once your baby is happily nursing on the breast, you really don't need to stop to burp your baby. Because of the tight latch a baby has on the breast, she will take in considerably less air than a baby feeding from a bottle. The only time I burp a nursing baby is if the baby gets sleepy on the breast and she hasn't eaten for a sufficient amount of time.

You may also interrupt the feeding to burp the baby if you have an abundance of milk and your baby is gulping down the milk. Then, pull her off to slow her down and slow down your milk production a little. Otherwise you just need to burp in between breasts and at the end of the feeding.

After you have fed and burped the baby, swaddle your baby and hold her for a little while to give time for the food to digest. Then, if your baby is sleepy, gently place her in her bassinet or crib. If she is awake and alert, this is a great time to talk to her, sing to her, or just walk around and show her where she lives—the kitchen, the pictures, the view from the window.

Don't keep her awake too long. As soon as she shows signs of being sleepy, she should be swaddled and put down to sleep. It is so important for your baby to get the sleep she needs for her brain development, as well as for her overall physical development. A rested baby is a happy baby!

7:30 P.M.	Feeding
10:00 P.M.	Feeding
1:00 A.M.	Feeding
4:00 A.M.	Feeding
7:00 A.M.	Feeding (starting next day's schedule)

If you are bottle-feeding, you should remain on a three-hour schedule. Though it's unlikely, if your baby is sleeping at night for more than three-hour stretches at a time, you don't have to wake him after three hours to feed. A formula-fed baby can go up to five hours without waking; you can see how much formula he is getting, as well as the fact that the formula takes longer to digest than breast milk. Note: *If you are bottle-feeding with breast milk, follow the breast-feeding schedule!*

SCHEDULE FOR BOTTLE-FED BABIES

7:00 A.M.	Bottle-feed. Unswaddle the baby and change the diaper. Burp well after each ½ ounce of milk and at the end of the feed.
10:00 A.M.	Bottle-feed
1:00 P.M.	Bottle-feed
4:00 P.M.	Bottle-feed
7:00 P.M.	Bottle-feed

10:00 P.M.   Bottle-feed

2:00 A.M.   Bottle-feed

6:00 A.M.   Bottle-feed

You will see that I put in two four-hour stretches, one at 10:00 P.M. (the Dream Feed) and the other at 2:00 A.M. Your baby may or may not sleep this long. Some babies are just a little sleepier than others, which can be caused by whether the mom is taking pain relief medication or not, how big the baby is, and how much he is drinking. This doesn't mean you should force your baby to drink as much as possible; overfeeding your baby can cause him to sleep less, as he will be gassier, possibly spit up more, and be generally uncomfortable. The amount he eats will depend on his stomach size!

But once you pass 6:00 A.M., you need to go back to feeding every three hours, no matter what. So initially there may be some fluctuation in sleep schedule, but the one time you always need to keep the same is the 10:00 P.M. feed, so adjust your baby's schedule a little so you can fit in that feeding. For example:

6:00 A.M.

9:15 A.M.

12:30 P.M.

3:45 P.M.

7:00 P.M.

10:00 P.M.

Here is another way the schedule can play out:

6:00 A.M.

8:45 A.M.

11:30 A.M.

1:45 P.M.

3:30 P.M.

7:15 P.M.

10:00 P.M.

You are probably getting the idea! However you work your baby's schedule, end the day with the 10:00 P.M. feeding. The timing of this feeding establishes the routine for what will become the Dream Feed, which will be the last feeding of the night to encourage sleeping straight until morning—but not yet! You have about four more weeks to go to reach that milestone!

IS YOUR BABY GETTING
ENOUGH TO EAT?

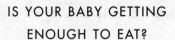

A rough guideline for how much milk your baby should be eating is two and a half times (in ounces) his body weight in one 24-hour period. So if your baby weighs 7 pounds, he should be drinking approximately 17 to 18 ounces a day. This translates to eight feedings at about 2 ounces per feeding. If your baby weighs 9 pounds, that translates to 22.5 ounces over the course of a day, which is about eight feedings of about 2.5 ounces each.

Some babies may be a little hungrier than others, but don't go too far over that 2- to 2.5-ounce feeding amount. Overfeeding can cause your baby to be extra gassy and uncomfortable, which in turn will make it difficult for him to settle down and rest. Overfeeding can also cause the baby to spit up more than he would normally!

If breast-feeding you can be assured that all is well if, at five days of age:

1. Your milk is in; the sign is mild to severe engorgement of the breasts.
2. You hear consistent infant swallowing at the breast.

3. The baby has at least six to eight very wet diapers per day.

4. Infant stools have turned yellow and follow most feedings.

5. The baby begins to self-wake for feedings every two to three hours.

6. The baby has eight to ten feedings per day.

7. Your baby seems content after nursing (relaxes at the breast after several minutes of nursing with active swallowing).

Remember, babies suck reflexively, so sucking does not always suggest that your baby is still hungry.

What if your baby is having trouble latching on? The number one rule is: FEED YOUR BABY. If you can express enough milk, you should give it to the baby in a bottle. If you are unable to express enough milk, then supplementing with formula is necessary. So, if your baby is not latching on, then you must pump at regular intervals (eight times per 24 hours) to maintain your milk supply until you can get assistance from a lactation consultant.

Managing Multiples

So how do you do all this with multiples?

If you are blessed with twins or triplets, it's definitely more work and it is even more important for you to keep your babies on a schedule. If you are breast-feeding, get advice from a lactation consultant on how to feed both at the same time. It's a little tricky at first, but once you master it, you will save yourself a lot of time.

Generally, if you're nursing two infants at once, do it on the bed, with a king-size soft pillow across your lap to support the babies. You can have both babies on the bed beside you. You pick up one baby, latch her on, then pick up the other one and latch him on. In the beginning, the first baby will probably lose her latch with all the movement, but just relatch her and carry on feeding.

If you are bottle feeding, you feed them both at the same time, either by yourself or with your husband or partner. You can feed both babies by putting them in bouncy seats, sit with one on either side of you, and hold their bottles. Or you could prop them on Boppy cushions or firm pillows. When you need to burp them, just pick up one at a time and burp him or her. If you are burping one and the other one gets fussy, don't feel stressed; just finish burping the baby you have, then you can get to the other one. With twins, one baby is usually fussier than the other, so I always recommend taking care of that one first.

(continued)

Managing Multiples (continued)

With triplets, it's a little trickier, as you can't breast-feed three at the same time! So, breast-feed two and bottle-feed one, alternating the one who gets the bottle each time. The easiest way is to have someone help you with every feeding. While you are breast-feeding, your helper can be feeding the third baby with the bottle.

Typically, multiples are born a little earlier than singletons (two to four weeks before the end of term) and tend to be smaller at birth. Often they will stay in the hospital a little longer, and quite often they don't come home until they reach two weeks old. This delay in sending triplets home is good for all involved, as the hospital will have your baby on a feeding schedule, making it easier for you to continue this routine when you bring your babies home.

LET'S TALK ABOUT CUES

By the second week, it's time to reinforce the cues to help your baby differentiate between night and day. At the 10:00 P.M. nightly feeding, keep your baby's room darker, with only as much light as you need to change her diaper before feeding, and then lower it further for the feeding. Obviously, you need to keep it at the level that won't put *you* to sleep!

From now on all night feedings should be done with absolute minimal talking and interaction with your baby. Remember, the more you stimulate your baby, the more she will want to interact with you . . . As much as you want to enjoy every precious moment with your new one, the middle of the night is not the time to do it. Eventually this will be sleeping time; now you are only up to feed. Any talking should be at a very low, calm level. One mother I worked for loved to turn on the TV and watch shows to keep her awake during the feedings. I advised her against it, but if this is the only thing that will keep you awake, then keep the volume down as much as possible. During the day, from the 7:00 A.M. feeding onward, all feeding should be done in as much light as possible. During these daytime feedings, you should also talk, sing, or make eye contact with your baby as much as possible. This interaction signals to your baby that it is daytime and you are happy for her to be alert.

I recently had a dad tell me that he had heard the first three months of the baby's life is considered the fourth trimester, and that your baby should be kept in a quiet semi-darkness the entire first three months, ideally with a sound machine running or with quiet, calming music. He explained that this approach would help ensure a calm, relaxed baby. This is a really nice theory, but it seems unrealistic. Don't we wish we could all have an environment like that, devoid of stress and outside influences? In the real world, we try to keep the baby's environment as calm and relaxed as possible, but instead of fitting our lives into the baby's world, we need to fit the baby's life into our world. This means that, during the day if you have a noisy house, you keep it that way. If you're used to a quiet and calm house, then your baby will adapt to this environment. Believe me, I have seen babies adjust and sleep through all sorts of chaos and noise. When you tiptoe around them, you just create super-sensitive light sleepers.

I once got a call from a mom whose three-month-old son would wake at the slightest noise in their house. The parents had tried to keep the house as quiet as possible at all times, from the moment he arrived and now he woke at every little sound! They had also established a few other bad habits. The mother had hired a baby nurse who would prop herself with about five pillows in a semi-upright position at night, and then the baby would happily sleep on her chest. Now, she was a rather buxom woman, so it was pretty comfortable for the little guy. The problem was that the mother had no chest at all, so not only was she left with a baby who wouldn't sleep in his crib but she had a baby who wouldn't settle on her somewhat flat chest. Add to the mix that the baby had to be walked up and down for half an hour to fall asleep, in a house that had to be kept as quiet as possible. This situation was quite a mess!

It took us a little while, but the baby eventually did learn to sleep in his crib—and with some noise in the house. During the transition, we added a white-sound machine to his room to try to help him sleep through the noise of the house, so that the house could return to normal once again, a recommendation I make only if absolutely necessary.

You can help your baby learn to recognize cues for eating and sleeping by using these cues consistently. For instance, when you always change your baby before a feeding, she will soon associate waking hungry with being changed, and she will know that she will soon be fed. If you have a baby who fusses because she doesn't like being changed, she will quickly learn to settle, as she knows the feeding is coming next.

Always placing a burp cloth or bib under your baby's chin is another important cue that his feeding is coming. I have seen a crying baby immediately become calm and open his mouth for a feeding as soon as the burp cloth was placed under his chin. Likewise, your baby will learn that being swaddled after the feeding is a cue to settle down and go back to sleep.

Babies thrive on consistency, so it's important that you keep to the same routine at feeding times. This doesn't mean you have to sit in the same chair, though some babies do seem to respond well to being fed in the same place (more or less) every time. But I do mean that you should try to get into the habit of changing the diaper, feeding the baby, burping her, and holding her after the feeding. You don't always have to swaddle straight after the feeding during the day; if your baby is awake then, let her stretch and interact with you a little. If you go through these steps in the same way, you will make your baby feel so much more safe and secure.

POOPS

By now, your baby's poops will be a yellow mustard-seed consistency, and if you are breast-feeding, they will be very frequent—in fact, your baby might have as many as three or four poops during one feeding. Usually, however, a breast-fed baby will have about eight to twelve poops a day.

A bottle-fed baby tends to have fewer poops, but should still be having four to six a day. It is possible for your baby to go a day without pooping. This only becomes a problem if she has a persistently swollen abdomen, in which case she may need some help—a little Vaseline on a Q-tip very gently pushed into her bottom can do wonders, as well as a warm bath. If you think that your baby is not pooping frequently enough, I would absolutely recommend speaking with your pediatrician. However, at two weeks old this really shouldn't be a problem.

You can also expect occasional changes in the color or consistency of the poop. It could be a little greenish, or seem a little runny, or even be a slight bit mucus-y. This is all normal, and related to the foods you are eating. However, if your baby's poop is black or there are any signs of blood in the poop, contact your pediatrician *immediately*.

If your baby has bright red blood in her poop, it could mean a few different things:

- Normal poop tinged with red blood is often a sign of a milk protein allergy.
- Constipated poop with a hint of red blood is probably the result of a tear in the anus or tiny hemorrhoids.
- Diarrhea mixed with red blood can indicate a bacterial infection.

Black blood can appear in a baby's diaper in little flecks that look like black poppy or sesame seeds. This is often because the baby is breast-fed and has swallowed some blood from mom's cracked and bleeding nipples. This doesn't pose a threat to your baby. Still, you should call the doctor to make sure it's not something more serious.

BREAST MILK

• • • • • •

In the second week, your breast milk should be regulating itself. Any engorgement should be subsiding, though you will feel fuller before a feeding and should feel a little less full after a feeding. If your baby has not been latching on properly, you will be feeling sore and possibly have cracked nipples. (See pages 96–100 in Chapter 4 for a description of the latching-on technique.)

If your baby is latching on properly, you should not experience cracked nipples, although they could still be a little sore. No matter what you and your husband have done pre-baby, I'm sure he wasn't sucking on your nipples every three hours, twenty-four hours a day, so they are going to feel a little tender! If your nipples are cracked, you may want to seek help with your latching-on technique from your lactation consultant, or ask your pediatrician's office for advice.

Amazingly, your breast milk may come in handy, as it has many healing properties. Try squeezing a little milk at the end of each feeding and wiping it around your nipple and letting it air-dry. Get as much air to your nipples as possible, as this will also help them heal. If your nipples continue to be painful, you may want to take a mild pain reliever, such as acetaminophen or ibuprofen, a half hour before a feeding. But as always, check with your doctor first.

WHAT'S GOING ON WITH YOUR BABY: WEEK TWO

GAS AND FOOD INTOLERANCES

Is your baby very gassy? This could be happening for a few different reasons. The easiest and most common reason is that the baby isn't burping enough. The air has to get out one way or another; if it doesn't come out, it will go down. Spend a little extra time burping, especially if you are bottle-feeding. The trick is not to hold your baby in one position to burp. Sit him on your lap to burp (keeping the baby's back nice and straight), then move him to your shoulder if you don't get a burp.

When you do move your baby to your shoulder,

let his body stretch a little; you want him to get accustomed to having a nice, straight back. This position allows the bubbles to easily rise in an upward movement. Sometimes one burp isn't enough, so don't start feeding again the moment you get the first burp. Give your little one a couple of minutes more to see if anything else happens.

Just remember that their little digestive systems are new and essentially they just need to work out all the kinks, so a certain amount of gas is normal and to be expected. Every baby handles gas differently, but the general rule is this: if you are calm, the baby will generally work through his discomfort in a calm manner; however, crying for more than half an hour at every feeding may be a sign that you need to check your diet or that your baby may not be tolerating well the formula you are using. Remember a little gas is normal, so don't change your diet every time your baby seems gassy. Consider removing foods from your diet only when your baby seems physically distressed or highly uncomfortable.

Serious gas can also be one of the first signs of dietary intolerances. If you are breast-feeding, think about what you are eating and how it may be affecting the baby through your breast milk. Many babies spit up a lot if the mom consumes a lot of dairy products. Again, a little spit up is normal; a lot of spit up isn't.

A general rule of thumb for a breast-feeding mom's diet is to eat small amounts of everything so it's a balanced diet. But be aware that if you have eaten something that gives *you* gas, then it is highly likely to cause gas in your baby.

Some of the foods you may want to avoid are:

Broccoli
Cauliflower
Beans
Sweet potatoes

Other intolerances can be more serious, especially if your new baby is allergic or intolerant to dairy products, including lactose (milk sugar) or casein (milk protein), gluten (wheat protein), and soy. It is always good to look at your direct family history to see if you or your husband (or other family members) have any allergies or intolerances.

Sometimes a baby with food intolerances may not show any signs of this initially. I worked for a family who hired me for the first two weeks after their baby came home. The little boy, who woke up every two and a half hours to feed would sleep peacefully in between feedings and showed no signs of any intolerances to lactose, dairy, or anything else that his mother was eating. Two days after I left, I got a call from the mom: "We don't know what we're doing

Formulas for Sensitive Babies

Many babies are sensitive to or have reactions to formulas based on cow's milk or soy. When you're looking for an alternative, know your options and check with your pediatrician first. Essentially, you will be looking for:

- Formulas made from proteins other than casein, such as whey, soy, and goat's milk
- Formulas made from casein that are pre-digested, such as Alimentum and Nutramigen
- Highly sophisticated formulas for severely reactive children that use free-form amino acids made in a laboratory, such as Neocate or EleCare

wrong! He doesn't settle, he's constantly crying, he seems gassy all the time, and he's started to spit up much more!" After going through all the obvious questions, I started to think that something else was going on. They didn't seem to have any allergies in the family, but nonetheless the baby's behavior was indicating allergies were the problem.

Over the next few months and after many visits to the pediatrician and specialists, they found out their little boy was allergic to many foods, including dairy, soy wheat, and eggs. Mom was put on a very restricted diet so she could continue breast-feeding, and introducing solid food brought a whole new set of issues—the family needed to have an epipen on hand at all times, in case the baby had a severe allergic reaction. While this was an extreme case, if your baby shows any signs of extreme discomfort, always discuss the possibility that he may have allergies with your pediatrician, especially if there is a history of allergies or intolerances in your family.

JAUNDICE CHECK-IN

If your baby had jaundice when he was born, you should start seeing a difference by the end of Week Two, as long as you have been putting your baby in indirect sunlight or under a phototherapy light. The jaundice starts in the eyes and slowly moves down the body, and when it starts to dissipate, it goes in the opposite direction. This means the eyes are always the last to go back to normal!

CHOKING AND GAGGING

Most babies at some point will choke a little on their milk, and this can be scary. When your baby chokes on the milk he is drinking, remember that as long as your baby is coughing and sounding like he is choking, then he is fine—he is clearing the milk or spitting it up from his throat. *Don't panic.* Lift your baby's arms, as this can help the milk go down. Sit your baby upright or put your hands under his arms and hold him straight up. In some cases, you may need to use the nose bulb and suction some of the excess milk from your baby's mouth, but this is rarely needed.

If you're bottle-feeding, gagging often occurs during the first couple of weeks, when you first put the bottle in your baby's mouth. The gag reflex should lessen over time, but some babies will have a stronger gag reflex than others; if your baby does gag frequently when you put the bottle in her mouth, then you are going to have to be a lot slower in your approach. First, gently rub the nipple on your baby's lip, letting her know it's coming. Then, wait until she shows that she wants it, and let her suck it into her mouth. Let the baby be your guide; don't push the bottle too far back in.

CORD CARE

Many parents wonder about how long their baby will have an umbilical cord stub and what they should do with it once it falls off. It typically takes ten to twenty-one days for the cord to dry up and drop off. Sometimes it can take a little longer. When it does drop off, it will leave a small wound that may take a few days to heal.

Beware the Witching Hour!

I'm sure you have heard horrible tales of a baby's witching hour—that testy time of day when babies struggle to shift from day to night. Many babies become cranky, irritable, seem hungry but are not, and are just downright difficult during the time between 5:00 and 7:00 P.M. As the day ends, your baby is getting a little more tired and ready to settle for the night, and this fussy period is just his way of letting you know how he feels. Sometimes a baby's fussiness is caused by a little build up of gas, if he hasn't gotten all his burps up throughout the day, and sometimes it is just tiredness (which may seem hard to believe when all he does is eat and sleep at this point).

Often, moms want to feed their babies at this time, but that doesn't necessarily stop the fussiness. In fact, sometimes it can make it worse, especially if your baby is a little gassy. This is a time when you may just need to hold your baby a little more. This can also be a good time to have the family over to also enjoy holding your baby, even if she is a little fussy.

While the cord is attached, it must be kept clean and dry. You should fold your baby's diaper over so it sits below the cord (or buy newborn diapers with a cut-out space for the cord) so it's exposed to the air and not to urine. When the cord falls off, you may detect a little blood on the diaper, which is normal.

Avoid giving your baby a full bath until this happens. It used to be recommended to keep the area around the cord clean by wiping around the base of the cord with alcohol. However, it is now *not* recommended to use alcohol. I suggest you have alcohol on hand, but only use it if the cord area becomes smelly, or there are clear signs of irritation. The best thing to do is to dip a cotton swab in the alcohol, wipe it gently around the base of the cord, and pat the area dry.

If you do suspect an infection because your baby has a fever and appears unwell, or if the navel and the surrounding area become swollen or red, or there is pus at the base of the cord, then you should contact your doctor immediately.

YOUR SECOND-WEEK DOCTOR VISIT

A t the end of the two weeks, your pediatrician will want to see you and your baby.

Before your doctor visit, it's a good idea to prepare the information your doctor will want to know about you and your baby. Here's a list of questions the doctor may ask; of course, if you are using your

Preemies

If your baby was born premature, don't follow my schedules for feeding and sleeping until you have been told it is okay to do so by your doctor. Your baby will have his own set of challenges to face, and if you're parenting a preemie, you'll need additional support and medical guidance on your baby's health, development, feeding, and care. Caring for a premature baby is different—preemies are more likely to have feeding problems, may have more trouble sleeping, and can be harder to soothe. They may also have continuing medical needs. Premature babies are amazing; they can grow and thrive despite huge obstacles, and they catch up to full-term babies in both size and development within the first year of life.

log, you may be recording these details and have them ready!

1. How is the baby doing overall?
2. Does she sleep regularly? About how many hours at night? During the day?
3. How frequently has the baby been eating?
4. How much does he eat? (If breast-feeding, you would measure this in terms of time per feeding.)

5. How many wet diapers a day?
6. How many soiled diapers a day?
7. Describe the poop.
8. Any rashes?
9. Any unusual behaviors?

You should use this time to ask any questions or express any concerns you may have. The doctor can tell you if your baby is progressing well in terms of height, weight, and head circumference.

At this visit your baby will be weighed; she should weigh as much as she did at birth, or more. This weight gain will let you know whether or not your baby is eating sufficiently. If your baby has reached that milestone, then you can begin to stretch out the time between feedings at night. If your baby has not reached her birth weight, then you should continue to feed her every two and a half to three hours.

BACK TO YOU, MOM

You may continue experiencing moderate to severe sweating at night time. This is normal, so please don't worry. One mom I worked for changed on average three times a night because her night clothes were saturated!

Your bleeding and discharge should have slowed down considerably by now. You may experience occasional heavy spotting; again, this is normal. The only time you need to be concerned is if you are passing very large, bright red clots. Then contact your doctor immediately.

By the end of Week Two, you may feel your energy levels decreasing. Some of the euphoria and excitement (some call it nervous energy!) has worn off, and the effects of interrupted sleep are taking their toll on you. Your baby is content sleeping and waking up every three hours or so. But that's not what you're used to!

If you have had too many visitors, this will start to really wear you out, so it's important for you to nap when your baby is sleeping. It will do you and your milk supply good. Remember: if you get too tired or stressed, or don't eat and drink sufficiently, this can affect your milk supply.

How much should you drink? The recommended amount is 8 ounces of liquid at every feeding. You want to drink plenty of water, plus some fruit juice and/or milk. Carbonated drinks aren't recommended, as they can cause the baby to have gas.

Many women ask me whether it's safe to drink
coffee while nursing. The good news is that one small
cup of coffee in the morning is fine—it won't be bad
for your baby. So enjoy, but make sure it is just one!
If you are a tea drinker, again try to stick to one cup
of caffeinated tea a day. Herbal or other noncaffein-
ated teas are fine to drink and enjoy.

To explain further, caffeine is a dangerous cul-
prit. When caffeine enters your bloodstream, a small
amount of it ends up in your breast milk. Your baby's
body isn't able to break down and remove the caffeine
very easily, especially in the first few months of life,
so over time it may accumulate in his system. Drinking more than two or three cups a day of a caffeinated
beverage may cause one or both of you to become irritable, jittery, or agitated and it can contribute to sleep
problems.

HEALTHY EATING, BREAST-FEEDING OR NOT
A mom taking care of a new baby needs her nutrition, especially if she is breast-feeding. This does not
mean you have to "eat for two," or give yourself free
rein to attack the ice cream and brownies. Sweets that
contain a lot of white sugar (like that in ice cream,
baked goods, and candy) are essentially "empty calories" for you and your little one.

I suggest a simple, easy-to-get-your-head-around

eating plan that enables you to eat most of your favorite foods and may just introduce you to some new foods that you have not had a chance to enjoy!

1. Eat a balance of whole grains, lean protein, and good-for-you fats (see box, page 160).
2. Drink plenty of water, up to eight 8-ounce glasses a day.
3. Don't go overboard on counting calories or adding calories; stay within 500 calories of what you normally would eat.
4. Keep taking your prenatal vitamins, as you need your vitamins C, D, and A, as well as calcium.
5. Avoid sweets and fatty desserts.
6. Eat plenty of fresh veggies and fruit (though as I mention above, cruciferous vegetables such as broccoli and cauliflower can make you gassy, which in turn will make your baby gassy).
7. Be moderate and mindful when enjoying alcohol. Having a glass of wine to relax may be beneficial, but alcohol in breast milk will be absorbed by your baby. If you do partake, make sure you express the milk within an hour of drinking the wine or beer, and discard the milk you express.

These are just guidelines to make sure you get all the nutrition that you need, whether you are breast-feeding or bottle-feeding. So don't go overboard on sweets and eat as close to the earth as possible—lots of grains, fruits, veggies, and lean proteins. You will see that the better you eat, the better you will feel—and so will baby! Here are menus for three sample days of healthful eating for a new mom:

DAY 1 _____

Breakfast	Whole-grain pancakes (sprinkle batter with a tablespoon of wheat germ) and then top with 1 tablespoon syrup or jam; cup of coffee or tea
Snack	Fruit smoothie with yogurt
Lunch	Green salad with grilled chicken and avocado
Snack	Cottage cheese with side of almonds and berries or banana
Dinner	Stir-fried chicken (or beef) and vegetable medley, including onions, red or green peppers, and zucchini or yellow squash over brown rice. If you don't enjoy beef or chicken, then try the vegetables over quinoa—it's a complete protein.

DAY 2 _____

Breakfast   Oatmeal with honey, syrup, berries
             or brown sugar; cup of coffee or tea

Snack   Handful of almonds and a banana
             or an apple

Lunch   Burger, no bun or a whole wheat
             bun (if you don't like red meat, go
             for a turkey or veggie burger), with
             a side of fruit salad

Snack   Side of hummus and whole-grain
             crackers

Dinner   Pasta primavera—pasta noodle of
             your choice with fresh, seasonal
             vegetables or experiment with
             combinations, including squash,
             peppers and onions, and canned
             tomatoes, eggplant, and a grilled
             chicken breast

DAY 3 _____

Breakfast   Cup of low-fat yogurt with $1/3$ cup
             granola; cup of coffee or tea

Snack   Peanut butter on top of Ezekiel
             toast

Lunch   Greek salad of romaine lettuce,
             olives, tomatoes, red onion,
             and feta cheese; topped with

	1 tablespoon of red wine vinegar and olive oil, or bottled dressing of your choice
Snack	Hard-boiled egg with a side of fruit
Dinner	Grilled salmon, chicken, or shrimp with rice pilaf and a side of grilled or steamed asparagus or zucchini

Healthy Food Guide

GOOD CARBS
Whole-grain breads
Whole-grain pita
Whole wheat tortilla
Ezekiel breads
Granola
Oatmeal

GOOD PROTEINS
Chicken
Lean beef
Lean pork
Fish (but be careful
  of those fish high in
  mercury, including
  swordfish, tuna, and
  other big fish)
Low-fat cheese

Low-fat cottage
  cheese
Yogurt
Eggs
Legumes (lentils,
  dried beans,
  hummus [though
  dried beans can
  make some women
  gassy])

GOOD FATS
Olive oil
Avocado
Peanut butter
Nut butters
Sunflower seeds

IF YOU JUST FOUND THIS BOOK . . .

If you have only arrived at CHERISH just now and your baby is older than two weeks, you may want to go back and read through Chapter 4 (Week One) and follow Week One's feeding and sleep schedule. Your baby may be eating less frequently than a one-week-old, and sleeping less, but what's important is that you set up the rhythm and routine of the schedule . . . I recommend you feed your baby every three hours during the day, not two and a half. If your baby is sleeping longer than three hours at night, do not wake him; wait until he wakes. However, if your baby is waking to eat more frequently than every three hours, make him wait the three hours, and do not feed him more frequently than that.

CHAPTER 6

WEEK THREE.
IT'S TIME TO SLEEP!

Now that the honeymoon is over, the news is both good and bad. On the one hand, some of the excitement has worn off and your feel-good hormones have begun to subside; on the other hand, your baby is much more likely to be on a predictable schedule, enabling you to get some seriously needed rest.

By Week Three, your sleepy baby is now much more alert and showing more interest in you as you approach or snuggle him. He should be awake a little more during the day. He will also probably look at you when you are changing his diaper, and stare at you as you speak to him and tell him what you are doing. At times, your baby may still look a bit cross-eyed; in the coming weeks, any sign of being cross-eyed will disappear. If it doesn't, you will want to check in with your pediatrician. At this age, babies' eyes are still not strong enough to focus, and the optimum distance for seeing an object clearly is between 8 and 15 inches. It's interesting that this distance corresponds to the distance between the mother's and child's faces while breast-feeding.

You will continue to reinforce the cues for feeding and sleeping, encouraging the baby to follow your schedule. It will help you establish a routine that will give you good, healthy one-on-one times, productive feeding times, and comfort in knowing you can have a little time for yourself.

ESTABLISHING A ROUTINE

By Week Three, it's time to start establishing the routine of eat, awake, and then sleep. It is very important for your baby to learn to fall asleep without the aid of food, from the breast or the bottle. There will definitely be times when your baby is so sleepy that this is unavoidable, but if it can be avoided, you need to try! At some feedings your baby may be so tired that it takes all the effort she has to finish the feeding and she will then fall asleep straight away. This is fine, as long as she isn't falling asleep at every feeding.

If your baby has fallen asleep at a feeding when this would normally be an awake time, try to burp him, and then place him down, unswaddled, on a flat surface, such as the sofa, the bed, his crib, bassinet, or changing table. Watch him as he awakens more fully—this can then be his alert time.

If the baby is lying on the sofa or bed, you need to stay beside him until he wakes so that he doesn't wiggle and fall off. Even though he is still little, a baby can lift his legs and swing them to one side, and the rest of his body will then roll with his legs. As your baby is awake more during the day, you can begin to transition him to feeding every three hours. Your baby will go from eight feedings a day to seven now.

SCHEDULE FOR BREAST-FED BABIES _____

1. At the 7:00 A.M. feeding, you unswaddle the baby and then change the diaper.

2. Nurse 15 to 20 minutes each side. Burp well in between breasts and after.

3. You may need to change your baby's diaper again after the feed, and sometime during the feed, as she will have frequent poops.

4. After you have fed and burped your baby,

hold her for a little while to allow the food to digest. You don't have to hold her up on your shoulder; you could have her sitting in your lap or just in your arms.

After the morning feeding, you will find your baby is at her most alert, so it's always a good play time. This is a great opportunity to make eye contact with your baby or talk to her. You don't have to talk baby talk, but raising and lowering the tone of your voice, or singing to her will captivate her. She may not be quite ready for too much eye contact yet, but it's a good time to try to engage her this way. When you see your baby making signs of becoming tired—yawning, getting fussy—swaddle her and then gently place your baby in her bassinet or crib.

Follow the same steps for each of the following feeds:

10:00 A.M.   Feeding; after this feeding your baby will be tired, so let her sleep.

1:00 P.M.   Feeding; after this feeding your baby may be ready for a little play time or may still be sleepy, so follow her cues.

4:00 P.M.   Feeding; after this feeding you should encourage playtime. This

will help get her ready for the
nighttime.

7:00 P.M.   Feeding; after this feeding you
should encourage your baby to
settle down and go to sleep.

10:00 P.M.   Feeding; remember that, at each
feeding through the night, the
room should be dimly lit and you
should use only a soft, quiet voice
when talking to your baby. Keep the

A Gentle Note About the Feeding Flow

When you first go in to feed your baby at 7:00 A.M.,
try to enter cheerfully, slowly unswaddle her, but don't
pick her up straight away; instead, talk to her and let her
know it's time to get up. After a few minutes, pick her up,
change her diaper, and start her feeding. This gradual
waking will help reinforce that she is safe even when you
are not in the room.

Keep in mind that your baby looks to you for signs of
how to react to situations. When you don't run to him and
fret over his waking, and instead arrive calmly and with
a smile on your face, you are signaling that all is okay.
He, in turn, will internalize this signal that he is okay.
This kind of positive interaction helps to anticipate times
when he may wake before his 7:00 A.M. feeding.

talking to a minimum. After this feeding, your baby should be put in her bed to sleep.

2:00 A.M. Feeding

5:00 A.M. Feeding; this can be a slightly shorter feeding, as you need to feed your baby again at 7:00 A.M.

If you are bottle-feeding your baby, your schedule is going to look pretty much the same as before:

SCHEDULE FOR BOTTLE-FED BABIES_____

7:00 A.M.   Bottle-feed

10:00 A.M.   Bottle-feed

1:00 P.M.   Bottle-feed

4:00 P.M.   Bottle-feed

7:00 P.M.   Bottle-feed

10:00 P.M.   Bottle-feed

2:00 A.M.   Bottle-feed

6:00 A.M.   Bottle-feed

Note: the 6:00 A.M. feeding will possibly have a little fluctuation. If your baby is awake and wants to eat at 6:00 A.M., then just feed him a little (that is, a small, 2-ounce bottle) to resettle him until 7:00 A.M., so that the 7:00 A.M. feed is a good, full feed.

The only difference in Week Three is that you can

now leave your baby to sleep as long as he is able after the 10:00 P.M. feeding, remembering to feed him every three hours during the day. If he has gained back all his weight, you can encourage him to sleep at least four or five hours at night by gently patting and shushing him, or reswaddling him. Pick him up only if he's crying and it's the only way to comfort him.

SCHEDULING REFINEMENTS

Keep in mind that there will be very slight variances in feeding times. For example, if your baby is hungry and wants to feed at 3:45 P.M., then don't wait till 4:00 P.M. If your baby is hungry, then she will be rooting around on anything that touches her lips and trying to suck. All your usual tricks to console her won't work, so just go ahead and feed her. A few minutes either side of the hour is fine—just try not to deviate by more than 20 minutes, so you can easily get back on track at the next feeding time.

Often, when your baby has woken a little earlier for one feeding, he will sleep a little longer at the next feed. However, if your baby is waking up early and seeming hungry at every feeding time, then he is not getting enough to eat. This is your cue to giving him a little more in his bottle or to make sure he is eating efficiently at the breast. If your baby is getting very sleepy at the breast, then take him off and wake him up and get him started again. This will ensure he eats enough.

Very occasionally, a larger baby (one who was born more than 8 pounds) may want a little more in the evenings; this too is okay—especially between the last two feedings of the day, which I call the "cluster feeds." In such cases, larger babies might eat at 7:00 P.M., want a little more at 8:00 P.M., and then top it off at 10:00 P.M. for their final feed. This is fine in the Weeks One through Three, but make sure that your baby can still settle after the extra feeding and that it does not interfere with having a good feeding at 10:00 P.M.

The only two feedings of the day that must remain consistent at this point are the 7:00 A.M. feed and the 10:00 P.M. feed. They establish the morning wake-up time and the last feeding of the night, which is how you start to encourage your baby to sleep through the night.

You will also notice that I have put an additional four-hour stretch between 10:00 P.M. and 2:00 A.M. If your baby should wake before 2:00 A.M., try to re-settle her rather than offering a feeding straight away. By resettling, I mean patting and shushing a little, or even reswaddling if necessary. Try not to pick her up unless you have to. I don't believe in letting your baby cry, so please pick her up if she starts to cry. If you can't hold her off until 2:00 A.M., then go ahead and feed her, but keep encouraging her to go a little longer each night between feeds. Gradually, she will.

SWADDLING

● ● ● ● ● ●

I f your baby is breaking out of the swaddle, don't jump to the conclusion that he doesn't like being swaddled; it simply means your baby is active! Many moms ask if it's still necessary to swaddle a baby at three weeks. I say yes! Swaddling keeps your baby's arms beside his body so he doesn't startle and it gives the baby a chance to get deep, restful sleep. Even if it appears that your baby will fight the swaddle initially, it is still a comforting feeling and is part of the routine when teaching your baby to sleep on a schedule. Your baby will associate the swaddling with sleeping time and it will help him to relax in anticipation of sleep. On waking, some babies will wiggle and get their arms free of the swaddle (obviously the tighter the swaddle, the less likely this will happen). But this doesn't mean that babies don't like the swaddle.

I worked with a baby girl who, at six weeks of age, started to sleep from 10:00 P.M. to 7:00 A.M. She did this consistently for five days and we thought, "Oh, great! She is now going through the night." Then she started to wake at 2:00 A.M. or sometimes at 4:00 A.M. Each time she woke early, she had worked at least one of her arms out of the swaddle.

Her dad kept saying to me, "Maybe she doesn't like the swaddle—maybe we should put her in a sleep sack." I explained to him it was *because* she was out of the swaddle that she was waking—that when the arm came out, it would be cold to the touch. I felt strongly that the baby definitely wasn't ready to sleep unswaddled. As a compromise, we switched from a regular baby blanket to the Miracle Blanket (a type of blanket that helps secure a baby's arms in place), which gave her a tighter swaddle. Straight away she went back to sleeping from 10:00 P.M. to 7:00 A.M. once again every night.

When the Moro (startle) reflex subsides at around four months, you will know it's time to transition your baby out of her swaddle. At that point, she will be able to sleep without constantly startling herself awake.

How Is Your Baby's Weight?

Babies who haven't gained back their birth weight have to be fed more frequently. You should consult with your pediatrician to understand precisely why your baby is not gaining properly. If you are breast-feeding, it's possible that your milk supply isn't as productive as needed—in which case, you may need to supplement with formula. There will be clear signs if this is the case, as your baby will be constantly fussy because of hunger. You can pump after every feeding to build up your milk supply or possibly supplement with formula.

If your baby is bottle-fed and not gaining weight, it's possible the baby isn't getting enough from the bottle. You may want to try a different nipple or bottle to increase flow. If you still have concerns, you should see your pediatrician for medical advice.

PACIFIERS AND NIGHTTIME SLEEPING

● ● ● ● ● ●

The use of pacifiers is a controversial topic. Some people swear by them and other people refuse to use them. All I can do is give you my point of view, based on my experience. I used pacifiers much more frequently in the beginning of my career, but now

Managing Multiples

If you have multiples, it is still important to feed the babies either at the same time or one straight after the other. You should be finding it much easier to feed and latch both babies at the same time now, but you may still need a little assistance. When one needs to be burped, you can just let the other one rest on the pillow and take turns burping. Then get them back to eating again.

With twins or triplets, it's very possible for the babies to be waking at slightly different times. If one baby wakes while the others are still sleeping soundly, try to settle the first baby back to sleep by patting and shushing or reswaddling. Only pick her up if she is crying. Don't worry that the crying from one will wake the other baby/babies—most newborns sleep through the noise of the other baby cries. If a baby wakens and really can't be resettled, then go ahead and feed her. Once she is fed, then wake the other baby/babies and feed them so that you keep everyone on the same schedule. By continually encouraging the first baby awake to sleep a little longer, he eventually won't wake so early. It's important for you to feed the babies all around the same time to limit the amount of time you are up at night and to keep the babies all on a similar schedule.

I try not to. I have come to believe that a pacifier is just a bad habit that covers up the real reason your baby is crying.

When your baby cries, she is communicating with you. She is letting you know she is tired, hungry, uncomfortable, or gassy, so if you constantly put a pacifier in your baby's mouth you can miss the subtle differences in her cries. If your baby is trying to let you know his diaper is dirty and you are putting the pacifier in his mouth, you're not actually resolving the problem. Your baby may go to sleep, but you are teaching him that you won't always tend to his needs; you just want him to be quiet!

Also, babies who are always put to sleep with a pacifier never actually master the skill of self-soothing. The moment they lose the pacifier, they are unable to get back to sleep. This means they will cry until you put the pacifiers back in their mouths, which isn't fun at 3:00 A.M., and then again at 3:20 A.M., and then again at 4:00 A.M. This sequence of events is inevitably what happens when your baby becomes habituated to the pacifier, as babies usually don't have the ability to keep it in their mouths. If you prop the pacifier in your baby's mouth so it doesn't fall out, your baby is then sucking on it constantly and never gets the opportunity to try to put herself to sleep!

So what is the alternative? In my opinion, it is simply to teach your child to go to sleep unaided. "So how do you do that?" I hear you asking.

When Is It Right to Pick up a Baby to Encourage Sleeping?

Any time the baby cries!

At three weeks or younger, no baby should be left alone to cry. It is not good for a baby's brain or nervous system. If, on the other hand, your baby is making little noises, you can try to leave her alone; if those noises get louder, then gently pat and shush.

If your baby starts to cry, pick her up. You can try to rock her back and forth and see if she will settle, but don't rock her till she is asleep; only rock her until she is calm and then put her back in her crib, patting and shushing her until she settles . . .

You may have to repeat these steps a couple of times before she settles. If she is rooting around and vigorously trying to suck on something, then she is hungry and you should feed her, but don't do this straight away—make an attempt to settle her first. Sometimes this is a little harder for a breast-feeding mom to do because, as soon as your baby smells the milk, she will turn to root! If you encourage your baby to wait a little longer before each nighttime feed, her tummy will eventually get used to going a little longer at night and so she will wake up less frequently.

Obviously every baby is an individual, so it all works a little differently and some babies will learn more quickly than others. But there is one unbreakable rule: hold your little darling for as long as you like, but when she is falling asleep, put her down in her crib right before she seems about to fall totally asleep in your arms. Your baby has just spent many hours throughout the day being held, cuddled, fed, and changed. You are signaling to her that it's time to go to sleep. When you put your baby down in her crib before she falls asleep, you are telling her that she is safe to go to sleep.

Of course, all rules have exceptions. If you have a severely colicky baby who can't be settled any other way, then I would use a pacifier. Occasionally, if you have a baby who is having a difficult time adjusting from the breast to a bottle, a pacifier can be used to help the transition. (This is done by offering the pacifier to your baby right before you put the bottle in his mouth, then offering the bottle. As the pacifier is a similar texture to the nipple, your baby will be more comfortable taking the bottle after the pacifier.) But always keep in mind that using the pacifier is habit forming, so the more you use it, the longer it will take to stop using it!

So when does nighttime begin? Ideally, it should begin after the 7:00 P.M. feeding. This should be a much quieter, relaxed time. Again, each baby varies and this could be your baby's "witching hour"! But even if this is the case, still try to keep it a quiet, relaxed time as much as possible. This might be a good time for dad to have a little quiet (not loud) interaction with your baby, a little snuggle time, a time for them to bond and interact.

WHERE IS YOUR BABY SLEEPING?

At night, you should really encourage your baby to sleep in his bassinet or crib. As tempting as it is to bring your little one into bed with you to settle, this can quickly become a bad habit. Sometimes you may be very sleepy at night, and it can be difficult to stay awake during the feeding, so you think "just this once!" But this is just the time when you need to pay attention to how *you* are feeling: you probably need to have more naptime during the day!

It is much better for you to feed and put your baby down, than to fall asleep with him and risk dropping him or his getting used to sleeping on you! I personally remember vividly that, after a middle-of-the-night feeding, I would wake up about 15 or 20 minutes later in panic, wondering where my son was, only to find him swaddled and sleeping peacefully in his crib. When I made myself nap during the day, I was more cognizant of putting him back to sleep.

WHAT TO DO WITH YOUR BABY
WHEN AWAKE

So, let's talk about the daytime. A common question I hear from parents is, "How and when do I play with my baby?" Playtime with your baby isn't complicated, nor should it go on for very long. Playtime in Week Three should be about a half an hour at a time.

At this age babies have simple needs. I usually like to establish a routine by which in the mornings after their feeding and digestion time, they have a little time on the floor. Simply put a thicker blanket on the floor and lay your baby on top. Babies love to hear your voice, so talk to him, sing to him, tell him what your plans are for the day. Just do it in a sweet, loving way. You can raise and lower the pitch of your voice, and he will be enthralled and just watch your lips move. You can even overemphasize the movement of your lips, and stick your tongue out a little.

Eventually, he will imitate you and start sticking his tongue out also.

This kind of interaction is important as babies begin to develop language. They need to learn how to move their tongues, and it is just the cutest thing to see them do it. You can also show babies simple, brightly colored toys, such as a little stuffed animal or a card of a picture with simple lines, or you could read a simple story showing your baby the pictures.

But please don't overdo it; babies this age need only one toy at a time. Move the toy back and forth a little and side to side; this will help to encourage tracking with his eyes; however, he will still have a little difficulty at three weeks, so don't move it too far away or too fast. As far as your child is concerned, once a toy is out of sight, it is gone and he is looking for the next thing, so to help encourage focus and concentration, keep the toy in his range of sight. Talk to him about the toy; make up a little story about it. "This is Daisy the little doll, and she wants to play with you today. Can you see her brown hair and big blue eyes?" Don't worry about sounding silly; your baby just wants to hear your voice. He really doesn't care what you say; he just cares about *how* you are talking to him—with warmth and love.

Around the third week, I also like to start

"tummy time," which is just like it sounds: placing your baby on his tummy to see the world from this point of view. This vantage point encourages the physical orientation toward crawling and helps develop muscle strength in the neck, core, and arms. But be prepared—this isn't always a baby's favorite activity. Most babies won't last more than a minute or two in the beginning. Although it's okay to let your baby fuss a little while on his tummy, you should not let him scream, cry, or get upset. You are simply trying to give your baby time to wiggle and get the feel of being able to move more freely. If after two minutes he seems done, then stop and try again later in the day.

Babies also love pictures; they respond best to clearly defined shapes and bold contrasts. You can use toys designed for this purpose, or books or pictures you already have in the house: it is great for eye coordination. Babies also love to look out of windows and at trees. In the third week, if you are getting a little stir-crazy in your house, you can start taking your baby outside into your garden, or for little walks in the neighborhood, dressed appropriately for the weather. You can also take your baby for a walk in a baby carrier or wrap. If it is cold outside, it's important to have your baby dressed appropriately, with a hat and socks. Your baby's extremities will get cold very quickly, as babies are unable to regulate their temperature so well. If it is warm outside, it is just as important not to overdress your baby! Also, if you are carrying your baby in a baby carrier, take into account the extra warmth for you and your baby that comes with the body contact. If you are out in the sun, always keep your baby's head covered and protected from the sun, but don't use sunscreen until your baby is six months.

Avoid letting other people touch your baby at this point. (Especially if you have a fall or winter baby, as it is cold and flu season). There will always be one person who wants to reach and touch your baby; just gently ask them not to. Better to offend someone than risk your baby's getting ill.

Given all the time your baby still needs to sleep, there probably won't be more than two times in a day right now when you will have playtime. The rest of the time your baby is awake will be for feedings and just sitting a little with you, or even walking around with you in the house.

Ideally, you want to establish a routine now of awake time in the morning after the 7:00 A.M. feeding, possibly having her awake for up to an hour and a half (that's from the start of the feeding). But don't make your baby miserable; if she is really tired or irritable, swaddle her and let her sleep. After the

10:00 A.M. feeding, you will find your little one will be sleepy, so once she is burped and changed, let her go back to sleep.

After the 1:00 P.M. feeding, you may find your little one to be either alert or sleepy; every baby can be a little different. If you have a particularly sleepy baby, he will probably go right back to sleep after this feeding also. If you have a baby who is a little more alert, then encourage him to play a little now, but not for more than an hour after the feeding. Then re-swaddle and put him down to sleep.

After the 4:00 P.M. feeding, you should encourage playtime again. This can be the same as the morning playtime. However, if you had playtime in the bedroom in the morning, have playtime in the living room in the afternoon, so your baby has a change in his environment.

Once you have reached the 7:00 P.M. feeding time, your baby's environment should be kept quiet and calm without too much stimulation. If your baby goes to sleep after this feeding, then put him down in his crib or bassinet, as this will lay down the routine for the beginning of the night. If your baby is awake and won't settle to sleep, that's not a problem. However, I would encourage quiet time so that he gradually gets the idea that this is time to sleep.

Any feeding after this should have as little

What You Should Have in Your Diaper Bag

If you are going on a short outing, you don't need too much, but you should be prepared in case you're away from home longer than you originally planned. Your bag should have the essentials: diapers (more than you think you'll need), wipes, and diaper cream. Always have a change of clothes—for both you and your baby; you never know when a diaper may leak or your baby may have unexpected spit-up. I recommend having an extra blanket and a burp cloth; if you're bottle-feeding, you may want to bring a bottle. If you are breast-feeding, you may want to bring an extra blanket to throw over you and the baby, for privacy.

stimulation as possible, which includes keeping your baby's sleeping area as dark and quiet as possible.

TIME FOR YOU:
ERRANDS AND EXERCISE

● ● ● ● ● ●

Not everyone has the luxury of staying home all day with her baby; most of us need to get out and about a little to run errands. I am commonly asked when it is a good time to do this. Should you go out during your baby's awake time or during his sleep time?

I am a firm believer in the notion that babies should fit into your life and not you into theirs. Having said that, you do need to take a few things into consideration. Ideally, it is better to be at home during feeding times: (1) especially if you are breastfeeding; and (2) because there isn't always a clean place to change your baby. So my preference is to go out during the baby's sleeping time. As the saying goes, "Sleeping like a baby" really means a baby will sleep anywhere! You can "wear" him in his carrier or bring him in his car seat along with you on whatever errand you need to do. However, I still wouldn't let anyone touch your baby or get too close yet!

WHAT'S GOING ON WITH YOUR BABY: WEEK THREE

• • • • • •

CRYING

The only way your baby knows to communicate is by crying, but you can communicate with him through your voice and your touch. He can now recognize your voice and pick it out among others. Your baby probably loves to be held, caressed, kissed, stroked, massaged, and carried. He may even make an "ah" sound when he hears your voice or sees your face, and he'll be eager to find you in a crowd.

There are generally five reasons your baby will cry now, so going through the checklist will help you figure what is wrong. They are (beginning with the most likely):

1. **HUNGER.** If you know its feeding time, then this is an obvious interpretation of your baby's cry. Likewise, if you have recently fed your baby, you can eliminate this as the cause of her crying.

2. **DIRTY DIAPER.** Most babies don't like feeling wet or soiled, so it's always good idea to check the diaper even if you've changed it recently.

3. **GAS OR TUMMY PAINS.** Every baby has gas—remember, their digestive system is brand-new and it has to work out the little kinks! I have noticed an increasing trend of new parents wanting to label their babies as colicky just because of a little gas. Gas can't always be avoided, but the easiest wasy to diminish gas is to make sure your baby has burped properly. Should you use over-the-counter gas aids? Honestly, unless your baby has such severe gas pains that you have spoken to your pediatrician about it, then I don't recommend these until your baby is six weeks old. Give the digestive system a chance to get working

without having to help it along. Again, I stress a little gas is completely normal and to be expected. Babies aren't used to relaxing their bowels when they need to poop; they tend to tense them, as they are not sure what is happening. This is why babies often poop when they are feeding, as this allows their little sphincter to relax. Although I appreciate that some babies are much gassier than others, don't be too quick to label your baby as colicky (colic is defined as inconsolable crying for three hours or more, at least three times a week for about a month). Try to figure out what is causing the gas first.

4. TIREDNESS. If you overstimulate, or try to keep a baby awake too much, she can get very fussy. Sometimes she just doesn't want to be held anymore, she just wants to be put down. Sometimes she will cry and/or fuss a little when she's put down. These little noises don't necessarily mean you have to pick her up again; instead, pat and shush her, and see if you can get her to settle in her bed. She probably will. However, if she is overtired, she will cry and fuss a lot more and it will take a lot more effort to settle her. You may need to put her down and then pick her up again a few times to get her to finally settle.

5. THE NEED TO BE HELD. Sometimes babies cry because they just need to be held a little longer. I do believe you can create a bad habit if you hold your baby

too much, but I don't believe in just letting your baby cry. So sometimes when you put your baby down and he is not quite ready, you will need to pick him up again. The most important thing is that you put the baby down right before he falls asleep, so he learns to go to sleep in his bassinet or crib without crying.

LIP BLISTERS

You may notice that your baby has a little blister on her top lip. This is normal and can happen because of the way a baby sucks when she's feeding; friction between her lips and the breast or bottle can cause blisters. These blisters tend to be more common in breast-fed babies than in bottle-fed babies. They are not painful, and you should just leave them alone. You may want to consider trying different positions while breast-feeding, but it isn't necessary; the blisters will slowly disappear on their own.

SPITTING UP

Many moms worry about whether the baby's spitting up is normal. The answer is: it depends. It's absolutely normal for babies to spit up a little after feedings. In fact, some babies spit up quite frequently and show no ill effects. If this describes your baby, then it's always good to keep a burp cloth on hand for these occasions.

However, if your baby is coughing or gagging during feedings or showing signs of abdominal pain, like arching his back, drawing up his legs, and waking up screaming, it is important to speak to your pediatrician. Your child may have gastro-esophogeal reflux disease and may need medication. It could also be the sign of allergies or intolerances.

There are strategies to minimize the spitting up. You can feed your baby in a more vertical position, so her back is straighter. You can also try to feed her smaller amounts and more frequently. In addition, you can try to keep your baby upright for at least twenty minutes after every feeding. I also recommend elevating the bassinet or crib at one end, so that the baby's head is always higher. Don't lay her down and change her diaper too quickly after a feeding; I recommend waiting at least twenty minutes.

UMBILICAL CORD

Most umbilical cords have dropped off by now. Once the cord has fallen off, you can give your baby his first real bath, twenty-four to forty-eight hours later. It's important to wait at least twenty-four hours after the cord drops off, to allow the belly button area to dry and heal.

YOUR BABY'S FIRST BATH

- - - - - -

At this stage, I like to give babies their baths every other night, before the 10:00 P.M. feeding. Most babies actually love being in the water and having the freedom to stretch their legs and slowly learn to kick and splash. However, be aware that the first few baths can be a little traumatic, as it's possible your baby may cry the whole way through the bath time. It will very quickly become one of your favorite times of day.

You should start the bath at around 9:45 P.M.; you bathe the baby and put him in his pajamas or a gown right before his 10:00 P.M. feeding, which will more than likely result in a nice, sleepy baby! The change in body temperature, from the warmth of the bath, helps to relax him.

Several years ago, I worked for a family where the father was a psychiatrist. His mother came for a visit and bitterly objected to my bathing the baby in the evening. Her argument was that the bath would wake the baby up too much and then she wouldn't relax and go to sleep. The father stepped in and said he agreed with me. In fact, he had recommended a bath at night for some of the very hyper children he worked with, and it did actually relax them so that they slept better.

HOW TO GIVE BABY A BATH

1. Choose a spot on a bathroom counter or kitchen counter that is secure and away from an open window or draft.

2. Assemble all the necessary bath accessories: towel, washcloths, baby shampoo, soft bristle brush, plastic cup for rinsing.

3. Fill the tub. I really like the bathtubs that have a hammock; it supports your baby and allows you to have two hands free. If you have a hammock, I recommend filling the tub until it reaches the hammock; this way your baby will be sitting in the water and so stays a little warmer. If you don't have a tub with a hammock, then fill your tub with about 2 to 3 inches of warm water. The water should be about about 90 degrees Fahrenheit (32 degrees Celsius).

4. Bring your baby to the bath area and undress him completely. Throughout the process, talk to your baby about what you're doing.

5. Gradually slip your baby into the tub, using one hand to support his neck and head, or if you are using the hammock tub, place your baby on the hammock. I like to wet a washcloth with the warm water and place it on the baby's tummy for a little extra warmth. Remember to rewet it frequently, as it will cool.

6. Always wash your baby's eyes first with either the washcloth or a cotton ball soaked in clear water and squeezed dry. Wipe his eyes from the inside out. Do not rewipe; use another cotton ball or a different part of the washcloth if you want to rewipe. Then wash the rest of his face, remembering to wipe behind his ears and under his chin.

7. Wash your baby's head with a little bit of shampoo and use the soft brush to help rub the soap in, using gentle circular motions. Rinse his hair thoroughly. This is the only soap you need at this time. You can then wash the rest of your baby with the water in the tub, from top to bottom, front to back, making sure you clean any rolls and creases. As for your baby's genitals, a routine washing is all that is needed.

8. Rinse your baby thoroughly with clean water.

9. Take your baby out of the tub and wrap him in a hooded towel. Pat him dry.

10. Apply Aquaphor to his diaper area. Diaper the baby and get him dressed.

The 10:00 P.M. feeding should be very quiet now, with dim lighting. This is the time I recommend starting to play quiet, relaxing music. You should play the same music every night from now on. It can be music you like, from lullabies to classical, but do bear in mind that whatever you choose, you will be listening to it every night from now until your child is two to three years old, so make sure it's music you like!!

Start the music playing as you are dressing your baby after her bath, or getting her dressed into her gown or pajamas before feeding her. The music should play for about an hour. This will give you enough time to feed and burp your baby, put her down to sleep, and still have a little music remaining for her to go to sleep with.

STIRRINGS IN THE NIGHT

B y now you should start to notice that, after that 10:00 P.M. feeding, you are beginning to get a little longer stretch of sleep. If your baby isn't sleeping more than three hours and starts to stir and fuss a little, don't go to her straight away. I use this rule: slowly count to 10 and you will often find your little one will be back asleep before you get to 10!

Obviously, this doesn't work if your baby wakes up screaming. Often, the scream isn't for food; it could be gas or a burp. In this case, try to pat the baby a little before picking her up, but if that doesn't work, pick her up and burp her a little. She may need a little reswaddling or just a shift of position, so turn her head a little to the opposite direction—sometimes this little shift can make all the difference.

After the 2:00 A.M. feeding, make sure your baby is burped well. You may need to offer encouragement to settle again before the 6:00 A.M. feeding. But remember that every 10 minutes you delay the feeding by encouraging your baby to sleep a little longer will reap you benefits in no time at all: your baby will very quickly stop waking so early and start to sleep longer and longer.

The most important thing to remember during the nighttime feedings is that there is *no* talking. When you first go into the nursery, you can very quietly say, "Hi, baby, it's still sleeping time, shush, shush." But no more than that. And remember that if your baby is sleeping, you go to sleep yourself! A rested parent is a better parent. No matter what you need to do, you can find time to do it the next day. If you have thank-you notes to write or e-mails to send, do it in the morning, not at night. Your baby is sleeping around fifteen to eighteen hours a day; you will find a spare moment. I have known some parents who find it hard to get back to sleep once they have been woken. If you are like this, you should still lay down and rest. Relaxing is just as important as sleeping; the tiredness will soon help you go back to sleep quickly.

WHAT ABOUT *YOU?*

. . . . . .

BREAST-FEEDING, MILK SUPPLY, AND PUMPING

If you are breast-feeding, you should be feeling more confident. You should be able to notice the difference between being full and not full. You may also be able to tell when your milk is coming in or is "let down." It's pretty amazing to feel your breasts fill with milk when your baby cries. Occasionally, you may feel it at the sound of any baby cry!

If your nipples are still sore or cracked at this point, you really do need to get some lactation help (see pages 96–97). You should also be well past the engorgement stage. If you are planning to go back to work in the near future, or you just want to build up a little extra supply of breast milk, this is the time to start pumping.

I always recommend pumping after the 7:00 A.M. feeding in the morning, when your milk is usually at its highest level of volume. Don't be concerned if you don't pump very much to begin with. Your baby is probably only eating somewhere around 2 ounces a feeding. The amount you pump should increase in time, and with consistency. I have known moms to pump as little as a ½ to 1 ounce at first, and after pumping consistently at the same time every day, the amount quickly doubled or tripled. I have also known some moms who pump a lot more, so don't be alarmed if you are a big producer of milk—this is a blessing. Overproduction is only an issue if you become extremely uncomfortable and your baby is having a hard time dealing with the flow of milk. Then you might want to consider reducing your supply a little (see pages 101–102). I once worked with a mom who would pump in the mornings and get 11 ounces of milk. This was in her third week. She was still engorged every morning because of this and her little boy struggled with the fast flow. We adjusted her supply a little by placing green cabbage leaves on her breast every morning for an hour, doing so for four days. It cut her milk supply down to about half, and she would only pump 6 ounces in the morning from then on. But it allowed her little boy to nurse a lot more easily and she was still able to store plenty of extra milk.

Pumping in the mornings can help increase your milk supply. Remember: breast milk works on a

Freezing Your Breast Milk

Freeze your milk in the smallest amounts your baby might take at a feeding, so if your baby is eating about 2 ounces, store the milk in 2-ounce amounts. Then your baby can be offered a little at a time to minimize waste. Do not refreeze thawed milk. Breast milk can be left at room temperature for up to six hours, refrigerated for five days, and stored in a regular freezer for three months. If you have a deep freezer (one that is not opened and shut on a daily basis), it can be stored for six months. Once frozen breast milk has been warmed, whatever hasn't been eaten needs to be discarded; it cannot be put in the refrigerator and reheated again.

Your milk is best placed in breast-milk storage bags or containers for the freezer. Bear in mind that containers will take up more space. Make sure you release the air from the bag so as to allow for expansion when freezing. The bags are less likely to break that way. I recommend laying the bags flat in the freezer so they take up less space.

Frozen milk can be thawed quickly and evenly under warm, never hot, running water. Don't thaw milk in a microwave because it may destroy nutrients and create hot spots that can burn your baby's mouth. You can also leave the frozen milk in the refrigerator overnight to thaw. Thawed, previously frozen milk can be kept in a refrigerator for twenty-four hours. Because cream separates and floats to the top, shake the milk gently to distribute the fat through the milk before feeding your baby.

supply-and-demand basis, so the more you demand, the better your supply. Other things that can help your milk supply include Mother's Milk tea, and the herbs blessed thistle and fenugreek. Ultimately, the most important thing is to eat well, drink plenty of water, and get enough rest. If you are lucky enough to have a plentiful supply, you can freeze the extra milk for later use.

Recovering from a C-Section

If you had a c-section, you should be feeling much better by Week Three, and much more comfortable moving around. However, since your hormone levels will start to drop now, be warned that you could cry at the drop of a hat. This is completely normal! Unfortunately, this is the week when sleep deprivation also starts to hit you. So if you feel a need to cry, just let it out. There is no point trying to be a martyr and holding it all in—all that emotion will come out eventually. My husband came home to find me bawling one afternoon, and all because his mother had fed to his brother the plate of food that my husband had left for me! All I had to do was put together something else, but, no, crying was the better option at the time.

IF YOU JUST FOUND THIS BOOK . . .

If you have just got to this book and your baby is three weeks old, you may not be ready to jump straight in; you may want to begin the program at Week One.

For instance, if you have a little one who is waking frequently at night, you will need to correct that situation before you can progress to the Week Three schedule. I recommend starting at Week One, and progressing a little quicker. It really won't take long at this point to turn your baby's nighttime awaking around, but it will take a little commitment. No matter how tired you may feel right now, a couple more sleepless nights may be necessary before you are able to correct your baby's habits. The good news is that your life will become much easier in the long run.

When your baby wakes at night, don't feed him just to put him back to sleep. Try to reswaddle, pat and shush, or as a last resort, pick him up and rock him. But try to encourage him to go back to sleep. Stretch his times between feedings to at least three hours. In most cases, doing this for two to three nights will be enough to adjust your baby's clock so he will stop waking so frequently. But it is important that he sleeps in his bed; if you do have to pick him up, don't rock him totally to sleep. When he is almost asleep, pop him back down and pat and shush him till he is almost asleep. Once this is done, you are ready to proceed from here, and put him on the feeding and sleeping schedule for Week Two. Again, you should be able to encourage your baby to sleep a little longer to catch up to the Week Two schedule and then you will be ready to carry on to Week Three.

CHAPTER 7

WEEK FOUR.
IT WORKS! THE PLAN IS
COMING TOGETHER

By Week Four, you should be well on your way to having a fairly consistent schedule. Your baby's nights should be getting a little longer, and you should be sleeping longer and better as well. With this kind of steady nighttime sleep, you should also notice that your baby's daytime schedule is becoming consistent and predictable. Yahoo! If this is not the case, you need to take a look at what could be going on.

By Week Four, many families start to notice the difference between their baby's progression and the way their friends' babies may be doing—none more so than a couple of dads whom I worked for who had twin girls. The one dad loved to go out on long walks with the girls and wrap them in a Moby wrap (a long piece of fabric that wraps around the adult while holding a baby). At four weeks, he would meet friends, many of whom were new parents as well, and he loved to share his good fortune about how well his girls were doing. For him, the fact that they were now only up once during the night was a reason for celebration—and a bit of gloating.

My favorite part was when he came home one day and told me how he was teaching a new mom friend of his how to wrap her baby and was giving her tips on how to get her baby sleeping better at night. After all, getting that little extra sleep makes such a world of difference when it comes to attitude and feeling confident as a parent—for the parent's well-being as well as the well-being of the baby.

WEEK FOUR SCHEDULE

● ● ● ● ● ●

This is the week that your baby is shifting from her sleepy self and becoming a little person. Her alert times will be more interactive, and her sleepy times will be more consistent. Whether you are breast-feeding or bottle-feeding, your baby's schedule this week should be pretty much the same.

This is also a good time to correct an old wives' tale: that a bottle-fed baby sleeps better than a breast-fed baby. That isn't true. If you have your baby on a good schedule and he is eating well, a breast-fed baby sleeps just as well as a bottle-fed baby.

This is how your baby's schedule should be looking now, whether you are breast-feeding or bottle-feeding:

7:00 A.M.	Feeding; awake until 9:00 A.M., then naptime until 10:00 A.M.
10:00 A.M.	Feeding, followed by a nap.
1:00 P.M.	Feeding, then awake until 2:00 P.M., then naptime until 4:00 P.M.
4:00 P.M.	Feeding; awake until 5:30 P.M.
5:30–6:30 P.M.	If your baby is still asleep at 6:30 P.M., then gently wake her.
6:45 P.M.	Bath time and change your baby into her night clothes; then start the nighttime going-to-bed music.
7:00 P.M.	Feeding, then put to sleep in her bed for the night.

It Works! The Plan Is Coming Together   203

WEEK
4

10:00 P.M.	Feeding; quietly pick your baby up and change her diaper; you may need to stir your little one for this feeding, but remember: it's worth it! If your baby is eating while sleeping that's fine, just encourage her to eat as much as she can. Little tickles under her chin can keep her eating, as well as pulling the bottle gently in and almost out of her mouth.
3:00 A.M.	Feeding; if your baby isn't awake at 3:00 A.M., let her sleep! Otherwise, after the feeding, burp her and put her back to sleep. No talking during this feed; it should be as quiet as possible.
7:00 A.M.	Feeding; good morning, baby! Even if she is still asleep, gently wake her.

IF YOUR BABY IS NOT FALLING
INTO A SCHEDULE

●●●●●●

Let's take a look at what could be interrupting your baby's feeding and sleeping schedule.

STILL HUNGRY?

Are you having a hard time keeping to the schedule? Perhaps your baby is waking up consistently early for his feeds. This could simply mean you need to feed him a little more. If you are bottle-feeding, add another ounce to each feeding and let him take as much as he would like. If you are breast-feeding, encourage your baby to eat a little more efficiently. When your baby is getting very sleepy at the breast, do whatever you can to keep him awake. It really is important to make each feeding time as productive as possible and you are now seeing why.

It is also important that your milk supply is well established. Do you feel that you have a full breast before each feeding? This can often be a little deceptive, as I have worked for a couple of moms who had a great milk supply but never actually "felt" full of milk. So don't panic if you don't feel the milk supply. The best thing to do is pump right before one of the feedings (preferably a morning one) and see how

It Works! The Plan Is Coming Together   205

WEEK
4

much milk you get. You won't necessarily get a large amount if you haven't pumped before, as your baby will always be more efficient than the pump; however, you should get a good ounce or two at this time.

If you are struggling to pump very little, then your baby may not be getting enough to eat; this will explain her fussiness and her waking early for each feeding. If you feel your milk supply isn't sufficient, then there are a few things you can do to help with the production; see pages 116–117 for some suggestions. The most important thing to remember is to relax!

You could also pump after every feeding. Pumping is time-consuming and can be a little draining, but it is also very effective. Ultimately, no remedies will work if you:

1. Don't eat enough. On average, a mother should have a daily diet of 2,500 to 2,800 calories.

2. Don't drink enough. I always recommend having a glass of water or juice at every feeding; if you feel thirsty between feedings, drink some more.

3. Are not getting enough rest. If you don't nap during the day and you get overtired, this will have an impact on your milk supply. Your body can only do so much!

4. Feel stressed. I have seen many moms lose
   good milk production because of stress.
   Relax, prioritize, and take care of you and
   your baby first. No one will care if your house
   is a bit messy or the laundry is not put away.

If you've tried to relax, have improved your diet, and have rested more during the day, and you are still not producing enough milk, then it might be time to supplement a little with formula. This is not the end of the world. Many babies have been raised happily and healthily on formula, and it hasn't affected their brain development.

GAS PAINS?

It could be that your baby is waking early because he is uncomfortable with gas. Remember to burp your baby thoroughly. Once you lay your baby down, any trapped air will move and this can wake your baby and cause gas or spit-up. If you have your baby on your shoulder and the burp won't come up, then change his position. I sometimes lay the baby flat on my lap, then pick him up again; this allows the trapped air to reposition and will often help bring the burp up quickly and easily. It's better to hold him a little longer and get the burps up than to put him down

It Works! The Plan Is Coming Together   207

WEEK
4

quickly, only to have him awaken again within the hour.

When a baby has gas pains, she will raise her legs and sometimes arch her back a little, and be showing all the signs of her discomfort. A baby will also root around and appear to be hungry, as the sucking can sometime relax her and allow the air to pass. If your baby has gas and you feed her more, then the gas can build up—or worse, it could cause her to spit up, by putting more milk on top of the air bubble.

To help your baby relax and relieve gas, you can first try to burp her some more. If this doesn't help, then lay your baby on her back and lift her legs up to her stomach, and push very gently on the bottoms of her feet. You can also rub her tummy; this provides a little warmth and can sometime help release the pressure.

Once your baby has released the air bubble, she will relax and be happy to wait until the next feeding. This applies to younger babies as well, but in the first couple of weeks, babies are less likely to experience built-up gas problems.

HOLDING TOO LONG?

If you're holding your baby until he is sound asleep, you are taking away his ability to put himself to sleep.

Don't get me wrong; babies definitely need to be held to feel the warmth and love from you. But they also need to be put down to sleep.

If you continue to hold him, he will get used to sleeping in an elevated position and will notice the difference straight away when you put him down. Also, he will become dependent on going to sleep in that position, as that is what you are teaching him. Then, when he wakes up, the only way he knows how to get back to sleep is by your picking him up and holding him. Not good.

Have you heard your friends say, "My baby sleeps so well when I hold him, but the moment I put him down he wakes up!" This will only get worse. I love hearing people quote that wonderful expression, "You can't spoil a baby in the first few months!" That's right—you can't spoil a baby. But you sure can teach him some really bad habits that you either will have to break at some point or live with!

My philosophy is, Why get to that point? If you teach your baby straight away how to put himself to sleep, then you have a happy, sleeping baby, child, and adult! So, let's go through the process one more time:

1. Right before your baby is fully asleep, you put him down in his crib or bassinet.

It Works! The Plan Is Coming Together   209

WEEK
4

2. If he fusses a little, then you pat and shush until he's quiet and drifting off to sleep.

3. When he is fully asleep, if you just can't contain yourself, you may pick him up and hold him a little while, but if he wakes up when you do this, then resist!

The most important interaction time with your baby is really when he is awake. He needs to see a happy, engaged parent, not an exhausted, stressed parent who is finding it hard to even smile!

FUSSING TOO MUCH?

Another temptation that can lead to bad habits is running to your baby's room with every little nighttime noise. At four weeks, your baby has become much more aware of her surroundings, and if you jump and react to every little noise, you could actually be disturbing her sleep cycle. Babies have a deep sleep cycle and a light sleep cycle; when they are in their light sleep, they often wiggle and make little noises. This is normal, and you are better off just watching, but leaving her alone. Otherwise, she will learn to wake at every light sleep cycle instead of getting herself back to her deeper sleep. As adults, our sleep cycles are very similar: if we are woken from a deep sleep, we are groggy and slowly come around.

Managing Multiples

It is just as easy to keep this schedule if you have more than one baby. Just keep in mind that your feeding times will be a little longer. The general rule with twins or triplets is to scoop them all up when the first baby wakes up. Don't let the others continue sleeping because you want all your babies on the same schedule.

It's quite common for one baby to wake a little more frequently than the other(s), so if you have one baby who consistently wakes much earlier than the other(s), then see if he will settle. Try to reswaddle or just pat and shush a little.

When I arrived to help one family with twins, the babies were already three weeks old. The parents were looking a little disheveled from lack of sleep. No one had suggested to them to have their babies on a schedule, and they certainly hadn't been told to feed the second baby when the first one was ready to eat. Consequently, they had two babies who were on different schedules, and the poor mom was trying to breast-feed them both, and never getting any down time. Just as she finished feeding one, the second one would wake, and when the second was done, within no time the first baby was up to feed again. I quickly taught the mom how to hold both babies so she could breast-feed both at the same time. Within a few short days, the babies were on a consistent schedule and feeding happily together. Mom was amazed at what a difference it made to her nighttime sleep and how it also allowed her to have a little more rest during the day!

It Works! The Plan Is Coming Together   211

WEEK
4

However, if we are woken from a light sleep, we can jump up and keep going for a while.

The bottom line? When your baby gets the sleep she really needs, she will be happier in every way. So this is a time to have your video monitor on if your baby is in another room sleeping so you can see what is going on, or just watch her without rushing over, so she can calmly get back to sleep.

CONSISTENCY BRINGS CALM

Keeping the schedule as consistent as possible calms and soothes your baby, as he then learns what to expect. It is important to anticipate and repeat how you do things with and for your baby; this repetition reinforces patterns of behavior and activity that, believe it or not, your baby also begins to anticipate and know. This regularity is what lays the foundation for your baby beginning to self-regulate and self-soothe.

Of course, as a professional baby nurse, I am paid to do nothing but care for the baby, or babies, in my charge, so sticking to a schedule is not a problem for me—I'm used to it. When you are a new mother who may have other children, a partner, and often a job as well, it's a challenge to juggle all those responsibilities and priorities, as well as your baby's schedule!

You should now be noticing the times when your baby is more awake than other times. For example, after the first feeding of the morning, your baby will be more awake than after the second feeding of the day. So make this a happy morning playtime. Open the curtains and say a cheerful "Good Morning!" as you tidy around his room or ready the changing table to get him dressed. When you approach his crib, smiling and attentively, unswaddle your baby but don't pick him up straight away. Let him stretch and be happy to lie in his crib for a few minutes.

If you always pick your baby up as soon as she wakes, she will expect this and learn to cry for you as soon as she awakes every morning. If, however, you create this new kind of morning-time ritual, you are allowing her the opportunity to get used to being in her crib or bassinet in a comfortable way. You are also laying down the first steps toward self-soothing—but more on that in a bit!

As he gets older, your baby will wake happily in the mornings, even before you go into his room. You might even hear him babble and play all on his own! This is a much nicer start to the day than having him always crying to get your attention immediately.

It Works! The Plan Is Coming Together   213

WEEK
4

SLEEPY TIME

After the 10:00 A.M. feeding, you will find that your baby is very sleepy and will probably either fall asleep during or go back to sleep straight after the feeding. This is to be expected, so simply swaddle her and put her down to sleep. This is a great time for you to shower, if you haven't already, or to get a little sleep yourself, if needed. Your little one will probably sleep all the way to the 1:00 P.M. feeding.

PLAYTIME

After the 1:00 P.M. feeding, you can expect a little alert time, but probably not for as long as the first morning awake time. Some sleepier babies will go back to sleep after this feeding also.

After the 4:00 P.M. feeding, you should encourage some awake time. This can last up until about 5:30 P.M., but not too much longer. Then put your baby back down to sleep. If you keep him up much longer than this, you could end up with an overtired and fussy baby.

THE WITCHING HOUR

As you probably have already experienced, the late afternoon–early evening has a tendency to be a fussier time of day for most babies, so it's important to watch

Learning to Live Through Your Baby's Fussiness

By now you should be finding that your baby is happier to drift off to sleep when placed in his crib or bassinet. There maybe a few times when he fusses a little before sleep, and that's all right. It is often the way your baby needs to settle himself.

I don't believe in allowing a baby to scream or cry himself to sleep at this age, so if your baby is struggling to settle, then some gentle reassuring pats or back rubs may help him settle. Obviously, if your baby is crying, then you may have to pick him up to resettle him before he will be able to get to sleep. The most important thing to remember is to not actually let your baby fall asleep in your arms, always putting him down right before he falls asleep.

Your consistency with this will pay off very quickly, as your baby learns to go to sleep by himself and that should help him sleep longer at nighttime. Your baby is very aware of your presence now, so if you run too quickly to check on him when he makes a noise, it will wake him unnecessarily. Use my Count-to-Ten Rule!

Of course, if you can tell his sound is more than just a little noise and it is escalating, then you need to attend to his needs. If you have tried everything and your baby is still crying, then pick him up and start the rocking and settling process again. But remember not to rock your

It Works! The Plan Is Coming Together   215

WEEK
4

baby totally to sleep; instead, settle him down and pop him back into bed. Occasionally you may have to do this a few times before your baby will settle, which is perfectly normal and to be expected.

This six-week period is what I call the "teaching period": you are *teaching* your baby to put himself to sleep. Sometimes he will settle straight away and sometimes he won't. But don't panic and think there is something else wrong. As long as you have gone through the checklist (see pages 208–209), he is probably just having a fussy period.

and make sure you don't keep up your baby for too long a stretch. Having a fussy period like this does not—and I stress does *not*—mean your baby has colic. Just as we come home from work at the end of the day and have a little grumble, babies also need to vent a bit. They may have slept more than half the day, but they still need to fuss and express themselves.

It is also important for your baby to have a little sleep time between the 4:00 P.M. and 7:00 P.M. feedings. I have seen several parents try to keep their baby awake to make sure she is sleepy by 7:00 P.M. Unfortunately, this strategy doesn't work with little ones, and it has the opposite effect. If a baby becomes overtired, she simply becomes more irritable and will have a harder time settling down to sleep. Just remind yourself of one of my favorite sayings: sleep begets sleep.

WHAT'S GOING ON WITH YOUR BABY: WEEK FOUR

● ● ● ● ● ●

BABY ACNE

Baby acne is a very common problem. It can be present at birth, but it is more likely to show up around the third or fourth week. You usually see it on the cheeks and sometimes on the forehead, chin, and even the back. The pimples will look like small whiteheads that might be surrounded by reddish skin. They can become more pronounced when your baby is hot or fussy, or if his skin is irritated by saliva or spit-up milk. Fabric that's a little rough or that's been washed in a strong detergent can also irritate your baby's skin, as well as perfumes and colognes.

Note: If the irritation looks more like a rash or more scaly than pimply, or it appears elsewhere on his body, your baby may have another condition, such as cradle cap (see pages 248–250) or eczema.

As with teenagers' acne, there's no clear explanation for the cause. It is often blamed on the hor-

It Works! The Plan Is Coming Together   217

WEEK
4

mones babies receive from their mother at the end of pregnancy, and certain medications that you may be taking while nursing, or certain medications that your baby may be taking can trigger baby acne. It is, however, important not to put creams or oil on your baby's skin, as this could make the acne worse. Just use a little water and mild soap and wash the area well once a day. The acne won't bother your baby so don't let it bother you. This acne usually clears up within a few weeks, but it can just linger. If it doesn't clear up within three months, or you're concerned about it, talk with your pediatrician.

Colic

Colic is used to describe uncontrollable crying in what seems like a healthy baby. If your baby is younger than five months old and she cries for more than three hours in a row on three or more days a week for at least three weeks (phew!), chances are she's colicky. Colic isn't a disease and it won't cause your baby any long-term harm, but it's a tough thing to go through for both babies and parents.

Colic can show up as early as two to three weeks, but typically appears around Week Four. Often, when your baby is showing colic-like symptoms at around two to three weeks, it may be a sign of some other distress, food intolerances, or digestives problems. A baby will cry for specific reasons, such as when she is tired, wet, hungry, or scared. But a baby with colic will just cry inconsolably and often at a similar time each day. If your baby has colic, you may see her pulling up and extending her legs and passing gas as she cries, and her tummy may look enlarged.

Colic is one of those great mysteries in a baby's life. About 20 percent of babies become colicky. The condition is equally common among both first-born and later-born, both boys and girls, and both breast-fed and formula-fed babies. No one knows why some babies are more prone to it than others; there may well be more than one reason. Your baby may have colic because his digestive system is a bit immature or sensitive. (In fact, the word *colic* comes from the Greek word *kolikos*, which roughly translates to "colon.") A newborn's digestive tract contains very few of the enzymes and digestive juices needed to break down food, so processing the proteins in breast milk or formula can lead to painful gas.

The act of screaming itself can cause your baby to swallow a lot of air and that, too, leads to gassiness. If your baby has colic because of tummy trouble, you may notice that his symptoms get worse after a feeding or before a bowel movement. Sometimes colic is blamed for the behavior of a sensitive baby who is being overstimulated and just can't handle any more

It Works! The Plan Is Coming Together   219

WEEK
4

sounds, sights, or sensations and thus cries to blow off steam.

Thankfully, colic doesn't last forever. Typically, it will peak at around six weeks and begin to lessen when your baby reaches three to four months. Your best coping strategy is to focus on what comforts your baby best. I once worked with a family who hired me for two days a week. I literally walked in the door at 10:00 A.M. and the mom handed me her little boy (who was usually screaming in discomfort from his colic) as she was walking out the door. My routine with him was to hold him in my arms, facing outward. I would walk over to the CD player and play his favorite CD. We would dance around the room like that for at least half an hour before he settled down. I would then try to play with him in his room or on a play mat until he started crying again.

We would then head straight back to the CD player and start the whole process all over again. He did sleep at nap times and eat at regular intervals, but most of his day unfolded in a cycle of sleep, play, and dancing—these were the activities that helped him relax the most. Our little routine calmed and settled the baby. Mom's days off gave her the reserves to cope the rest of the week when she was alone with the baby.

If you think your baby may have colic, then it's important to talk to your doctor about your baby's crying so that other potential causes, like intestinal or urinary infections, can be ruled out. If your baby should ever have symptoms like vomiting, fever, or bloody stools, call the doctor *immediately*. These symptoms are *not* due to colic.

Some breast-fed babies seem colicky because of something their mothers may have eaten. Although many foods are suspected of causing problems, dairy products are usually the most common culprits. If you're breast-feeding, try cutting back on milk, cheese, and yogurt for a couple of weeks to see whether that makes a difference. It is possible for cow's milk protein to remain in breast milk that long.

Other typical gas-inducing foods are spicy foods, wheat products, nuts, strawberries, cruciferous vegetables (such as cabbage, broccoli, and cauliflower), garlic, caffeine, and alcohol. Try avoiding all of these foods for a few days together to see if there's any difference to your baby. Then try reintroducing each separately to see if your baby reacts to any of them. But allow at least a day or two in between introductions of the new food. If your baby starts to fuss again after you start eating a certain food, you know to avoid that food until your baby is a little older. Of course, kicking coffee or any other food for a few months is a small price to pay for a happy baby.

Keep in mind, too, that your milk supply tends

It Works! The Plan Is Coming Together   221

WEEK
4

to decrease as the day goes on. By late afternoon you may be producing less milk than in the morning. If your baby is a bit fussy, it may be because she has to work harder to get the milk!

GETTING YOUR BABY BACK TO THE NORMAL ROUTINE AFTER ILLNESS OR TRAVEL

Although it's very rare for young babies (one to four weeks old) to get sick, it does happen. When a young baby gets a cold, flu, or just about any other illness, his sleep pattern and normal routine will be disrupted. Don't fret. Although many parents struggle to get their babies sleeping soundly again, there are some ways that put everyone back on a schedule—including you.

Obviously, if you have a sick baby, you have to attend to him night and day. You may need to monitor his temperature if he has been running a fever, and go to him every time he cries out, at night or during the day. But once he is well again, you have to go back to having him sleep through the night. This can be done very quickly and effectively.

Once you know your baby is well, if he continues

to wake at night, you will have to be a little firm and stop picking him up. When he first wakes, try the Count-to-Ten Rule before you go into his room. If he doesn't settle after that, then go to him and just pat and shush him while he is in his crib—*without* picking him up. Even if he is getting upset, do not talk or try to stimulate him in any way; just simply pat and shush him until he settles down to sleep.

Every baby will respond differently. Some will settle quickly and some may take a couple of nights to fall back into the routine. Try to be patient. Usually, it takes just two nights before a baby is sleeping through the night again. Remember: consistency is key here.

TRAVELING WITH YOUR BABY

Travel with your new baby can be a daunting thought! Your desire to get out and about, to take your newborn to visit friends or grandparents or other family members, can get very strong. Then there are the unavoidable pediatrician visits for exams, vaccinations, and other medical events. Although minimizing travel during the first three

It Works! The Plan Is Coming Together   223

WEEK
4

months is required, whenever you choose to travel with your newborn there are a few things to keep in mind.

Make sure the diaper bag is packed with all of your essentials. You'll want a supply of diapers, wipes, and diaper rash cream, and a bag for soiled diapers. You should always have a couple of burp cloths, and I always pack an extra blanket and at least one set of extra clothes, including layering clothes in case the temperature changes. And you never know when your baby's soiled diaper will leak through everything! The extra blanket can come in handy in keeping the sun off your baby; in the first few months, babies shouldn't have sunscreen on. In fact, the extra blanket has multiple uses; if you need to breast-feed, it will also come in handy to give you some privacy. These are the bare essentials.

Longer travel needs to be more carefully planned. Always check with your pediatrician before traveling with your newborn. I have traveled with a baby as young as four days old. This was out of necessity, as the baby had been born by surrogate in another state. The only reason we did it at such a young age was that we flew privately, and so the new baby wasn't exposed to all the germs and recycled air of a commercial flight. Sometimes circumstances will dictate a need to travel when your baby is very young, but it is much better to wait until your baby is at least three months old and has had his first round of shots.

Traveling to a different time zone can also be very disruptive to a baby's sleeping routine. Should you keep your baby on your time zone, so she is either up late at night or awake very early in the morning? There are two factors to consider when deciding how to handle the time change. If you are going on a short trip and the time difference is just a couple of hours, then you are probably best keeping your baby on his home time. So, for example, if you live in Los Angeles and you are having an extended weekend in Chicago, put your baby to bed at 7:00 P.M. LA time. Obviously, you will have to take into consideration that your baby will be up until 9:00 P.M. Chicago time and will more than likely sleep until 9:00 A.M. Likewise, if you are traveling from New York to Colorado for a short trip, be prepared to put your baby to bed at 5:00 P.M., knowing that he will be awake at 5:00 A.M. Short trips mean less disruption.

However, if you are going on a longer trip—one of a week or more—I would recommend adjusting your baby to the new time zone as quickly as possible. So, if you are traveling from Seattle to New York, the first morning you are in New York, start waking your baby close to 7:00 A.M. to adjust her to the local time.

It Works! The Plan Is Coming Together   225

WEEK
4

She may not be quite ready to sleep at 7:00 P.M. local time the first night, but she will adjust to it in about two days.

When traveling from east to west, you need to keep your baby up a little later each day and encourage her to sleep a little later each morning by not going to her too quickly. When traveling from west to east, you wake your baby at the normal home time of 7:00 A.M. and encourage her to go to bed as close to 7:00 P.M. as possible. Once you return home, you will need to get her back on her normal routine in the same manner. Either way, if your baby is having trouble settling, it's best to follow the advice on pages 221–222 after an illness.

WHAT ABOUT *YOU?*

By Week Four you should be feeling much better physically, and your episiotomy or c-section should be healed. Emotionally, right now you can still be very weepy, and this is normal, too. You can also be a scatterbrain, or have what we refer to as having "new mommy brain." I have been around hundreds of moms, and this is completely normal! You may simply need to write notes to yourself to help you remember appointments, grocery lists, or questions for your pediatrician.

Week Four can also be a big turning point when it comes to bonding with your new baby. What do I mean by bonding? *Bonding* is the two-way connection that you and your baby build together: each time you pick up your baby, feed her, hold her, change her, swaddle and unswaddle her, you are meeting her needs and communicating to her that you love her. As long as you attend to your baby's needs and kiss and snuggle her on a regular basis, she will feel loved. Human babies are born the most helpless of all animals, so they have a strong instinct to attach to the person tending to their needs. After all, you are your baby's only means of survival.

But if you don't feel that strong, all-consuming bond straight away, don't worry. There is so much emphasis today put on the mother-baby bond that some parents feel overwhelmed with nervousness and guilt when they don't know how to feel toward their child. The mom of one family I worked with was extremely happy with her baby, but finally admitted to me that that she resented her baby a little—there had been so much pressure to breast-feed frequently and she was so tired. The moment we established a better feeding routine, whereby she got a little more down

It Works! The Plan Is Coming Together   227

WEEK
4

time and rest, she said she had so much more love for her baby and less resentment.

One mother I was helping had quite a hard time becoming comfortable with breast-feeding. She had a very difficult time getting the baby to latch on, which frustrated her and also the baby. By Week Two, this mom was ready to call it quits and give up nursing altogether. I reassured her that it was possible to learn to breast-feed more comfortably, but first she needed to relax.

"Easier said than done," she said.

We then worked on ways to help her to relax. I showed her how to take deep breaths and to watch a favorite TV show or listen to music before settling into a chair to breast-feed her baby. I also pointed out that all that was required of her was that she should do the best she could—and that might mean deciding not to breast-feed.

In Week Four, she turned to me one day and said, "I hate to admit this, but I am only now enjoying being with my baby." The whole issue of breast-feeding was not allowing her to connect with her baby in a positive way, and now that she was able to relax and actually enjoy nursing, she was able to appreciate everything else that her baby was doing.

You can't force yourself to bond with your baby,

but over time and with the care and attention you give to your baby, that bond will form. When your baby starts to smile and coo at you, believe me, your heart will melt—and this is true for biological *or* adoptive parents.

TIME TO WEAN . . . OR NOT

'**ve talked a lot about feeding and sleeping, but what about weaning? How long should you breast-feed and/or how long should your baby have formula?

The formula question is an easy one to answer: your baby should be drinking formula until she is at least twelve months old. As I mentioned before, this is a baby's primary nutrition and his digestive system is not ready for any other type of milk until twelve months.

But when is the right time for you to wean your baby off of breast milk? This is purely a personal thing. The American Academy of Pediatrics recommends breast-feeding for at least the first six months, but not every mother can do it for this long, while some moms are happy to breast-feed for much longer. The bottom line is this: breast-feed for as long as it works or feels good for you.

It Works! The Plan Is Coming Together   229

WEEK
4

In the first month, your baby gets most of her immunities from the colostrum, before the breast milk is let down. By three months, she definitely has gained all the immunities that breast milk has to offer, and from then on it becomes nutrition. Granted, breast milk is considered the best nutrition for babies, but formula these days is so much more advanced than it used to be. So, if for any reason you don't feel that breast-feeding is for you, don't feel bad about it. There has been so much pressure put on moms to breast-feed nowadays, with promises that your child will be smarter or she won't get sick, that this stress alone can hinder a mother's ability to breast-feed well.

Do the best you can, for as long as you can, and be at peace with whatever decision you make. As I always tell my moms, "I was bottle-fed from two weeks old, as my mother didn't have enough milk to feed me and I was always hungry. I don't think I turned out too badly, although some may say differently!"

When you are ready to stop breast-feeding, it's always best to wean slowly, eliminating one feeding at a time. I recommend replacing the midday feedings first, substituting bottles of formula, then the morning feeding. The last feeding to be replaced with the bottle should be the evening feeding. Give yourself at least three days before dropping the next feeding;

this will give your breasts a little time to adjust to the lower demand for milk. If you find you are getting engorged, there a few things you should do and not do.

- You *should not* pump: pumping will just keep your milk supply going.
- You *should not* express or breast-feed for relief: again, this will keep your supply going.
- You *should not* bind your breasts: it used to be suggested that wearing two tight sports tops or binding your breasts tightly would help stop milk production, but it has since been found that this doesn't help at all and can, in fact, cause mastitis, a breast infection.
- You *should* use ice: if you have any discomfort from any engorgement, use a cold compress for relief—a pack of frozen peas works wonders.
- You *should* use cabbage leaves: as I mentioned earlier, placing green cabbage leaves in your bra around your breast will help dry your milk much quicker; replace the leaves frequently, and they are best when taken from the refrigerator—the cold leaves can feel just as good as the ice packs.

It Works! The Plan Is Coming Together   231

WEEK
4

If you need to stop breast-feeding quickly, then definitely use the cabbage leaves all day and all night, changing them as frequently as you can. If you need some extra relief, use the cold ice packs. If you have any problems, or spike a fever at any time, contact your doctor, as you may have an infection and need medication. Any clogged ducts that you may be able to feel can be massaged to relieve the lumps.

Whether you decide to continue breast-feeding or to wean, the most important thing is to enjoy your baby. Because, as we all know, babies grow up very fast these days, and then there's a whole different set of rules you need to know!

CHAPTER 8

WEEK FIVE.
HELL WEEK

f Week Two is akin to a honeymoon, then Week Five
is what a dear friend of mine calls "hell week."

Moms who have not yet been able to get their
babies on a consistent sleep and feeding schedule
will more than likely be hitting the proverbial wall.
You're run down, physically and mentally exhausted,
and feeling emotionally vulnerable and fragile—all
because you have not gotten the proper amount of
rest. The baby is probably doing just fine—more than
likely because he is getting plenty to eat and is sleeping adequately. But you have adapted yourself to his
schedule rather than vice versa. If things continue in

this way, even your little bundle of joy will begin to show signs of really needing to be put on a schedule.

This Week Five tipping point is the result of the sleepless nights finally catching up with you. Your hormones are stabilizing, but you are still very emotional—easily upset and stressed. Any family members who have come to help are probably slowly getting back to their own lives, leaving you in charge. This can be a time when the postpartum blues (or in more serious cases, depression) may start to kick in, so if you are having too many overwhelming feelings, you should talk to your partner or doctor.

One bonus in all this is that first little smile about to happen at any moment. There is nothing like a first smile from your baby to make all your aches and pains disappear. By Week Five, you may also be hearing an uptick in the little cooing noises—no doubt that, too, will lift your spirits.

If you have been following my week-by-week schedule, you shouldn't be feeling so overwhelmed or exhausted. Perhaps you don't want to run a marathon, but you should be feeling a bit more on an even keel.

What's the big difference?

It's more than likely that your baby is sleeping from the 10:00 P.M. Dream Feed to at least 4:00 A.M. by now, and you, therefore, have a lot more consistent sleep, especially if your partner does some of the middle-of-the-night feeds. This is still possible if you are breast-feeding. You can get up and pump, then let your partner or husband do the feeding. You should be able to pump both breasts at the same time, and so be done within twenty minutes and be able to go back to sleep. Or, if you've been able to accumulate enough milk by pumping during the day, you can use that milk in a midnight bottle.

Some doctors and other moms may tell you that a baby who is both breast- and bottle-fed will have "nipple confusion"; I can say that most women—and their babies—don't experience this situation. I have worked with many families in which the mom breast-feeds and I give the baby a bottle, either in the night or at the 10:00 P.M. feeding so mom can get some more sleep. I have not had one instance of nipple confusion. Now, having said that, if you have a very slow or low milk supply in your breasts, there are babies who prefer the bottle because they get more milk faster. This is not "nipple confusion"; it's a case of a baby's preferring the faster-flowing bottle. If you sense that your baby seems to prefer the faster flow of the bottle, you may want to limit the bottles, or pump and bottle-feed, but the first option is the best. Your baby may prefer one or the other, but with consistency and routine, most babies will follow your lead.

IF YOU JUST FOUND THIS BOOK . . .

For those of you who are just coming to this book, and you and your baby are not on a schedule yet, please don't worry: it's no surprise that you are feeling exhausted, overwhelmed, and possibly close to your wits' end! But do not despair! It's not at all too late to put your baby on a healthy, calm schedule so both of you can get some much-needed rest. If your baby is five weeks old, you will need to start at Week One. Once your baby is accustomed to the feeding and sleeping schedule described in Week One (Chapter Four), then you can go through each week at a faster pace, giving your baby a couple of days for each phase, and she should catch up very quickly.

YOUR BABY AT FIVE WEEKS

At five weeks, babies are much more interested in their surroundings. Your baby is ever more alert, and you will notice signs of his growing awareness of

you and the world around him. Here's a quick overview of what to look for at this time:

- Your baby should be close to smiling. Some
  babies will already be smiling at this point.
- Your baby's vision has improved. She should
  be able to consistently track a toy as you move
  it slowly from side to side.
- Your baby will probably look in the
  direction of sounds and voices (especially

A Little Extra Help

One of my fellow nanny friends has this piece of advice:
if you can only afford one or two weeks of help in the
form of a baby nurse, then Week Five should be your
choice. Why? Because if your baby is not on a schedule
yet, you will be absolutely exhausted by this point! The
endorphins and postpregnancy hormones will have
begun to subside, lessening your overall energy and
excitement. If your baby is still waking up every two
to three hours for a feeding, then you are going to be
completely exhausted and sleep deprived.

If you decide you want a little help, ask friends if
they have used anyone, or check with your pediatrician
for a recommendation. A local doula association might

yours!) and show a positive response to
your presence.

IT'S NAPTIME!

B y now you should be noticing some more consistency in your baby's daytime naps. You will see
that he is awake longer after the 7:00 A.M. feeding

be a good source of recommendations, too. Often, the
place where you purchase your breast pump and nursing
supplies may know of people who can help you with feeding
support.

You may also consider contacting a local nanny agency,
but do bear in mind that this kind of service involves a
placement fee. When considering a nanny, you want
someone who has helped with newborns and has experience
in getting your baby on a good sleeping and feeding routine,
not just another pair of arms for holding your baby at night!

But remember, even if you are not in the position to
hire help (or simply do not wish to do so), there is plenty
you can do to get your baby on a steady eating and sleeping
schedule so you will feel better very soon.

and is sleepier after the 10:00 A.M. feeding. This is the time to really start developing a good, solid nap-time schedule. The yawn is the most immediate sign that your baby is ready for a nap. But that doesn't mean that the first time you see a yawn, you pop your baby into bed. Time is also an issue. If you are within twenty minutes of the time he is due to take a nap, then that first yawn indicates he is getting ready. When you see the second yawn, you definitely want to start getting him ready. Change his diaper and get him swaddled. Always tell your baby that it is nap-time; you may want to rock him a little, but before he is totally asleep, put him down.

But it's also not a good idea to keep your baby awake too long; doing so can actually have the opposite effect. Your baby will get overstimulated, over-tired, and cranky, and will have a harder time settling down. So, how do you determine when to put your baby down for a nap? Look for the cues:

- Your baby will start to yawn.
- Her eyes will look a bit glazed.
- She will seem extra fussy.
- She will lose interest in people and toys.

I have included nap times in this week's schedule. This does not mean you have to follow this sched-ule rigidly, however. The feeding schedule should be followed as closely as possible; the nap schedule is a guideline only, and you will find you need to adjust it a little to suit your baby's sleeping needs.

Some babies at five weeks may not have as much awake or alert time, so if you find your baby is ready to sleep at 8:00 A.M. instead of 8:30 A.M., then put him to sleep. You can try to keep him up until 8:15 A.M., but if he is too sleepy, let him go to sleep at 8:00 A.M.

WEEK FIVE SCHEDULE, INCLUDING NAPS

• • • • • •

This schedule applies to both breast-fed and bottle-fed babies.

7:00 A.M.	Feeding, followed by playtime, including some tummy time; don't put your baby on his tummy until at least 20 minutes after his feeding is over.
8:30 A.M.	Nap.
10:00 A.M.	Feeding, followed by a shorter awake period, during which you may just hold and talk to your baby, with a little social interaction and not playtime.

11:00 A.M.	Nap.
1:00 P.M.	Feeding, followed by playtime and tummy time during this awake period; again, don't put your baby on his tummy until at least 20 minutes after his feeding.
2:30 P.M.	Nap.
4:00 P.M.	Feeding, followed by a little playtime and social time.
5:00–6:00 P.M.	Nap.
6:00 P.M.	Wake your baby if he has not woken on his own; do this gently and slowly.
6:45 P.M.	Bath time, followed by a massage, change into night clothes, and nighttime music. I tend to wait until a baby is about a month old before I start the massage after the bath; before this time, babies are usually too fussy to enjoy it, as they are usually hungry and don't want to wait for their food.
7:00 P.M.	Feeding, burping, then straight down to bed.

10:00 P.M.   Dream Feed; by this time, your
                    baby should be ready for a
                    good feeding and then be put
                    down before he is asleep in
                    his bassinet or crib.

4:00 A.M.   Feeding, burping, and back to
                    sleep.

7:00 A.M.   Feeding; good morning time!

THE FLOW OF WEEK FIVE

This nap schedule gives your baby more than enough time to be awake. Although I have mentioned the need for some flexibility with your baby's naptime schedule, your baby shouldn't be kept awake much more than an hour and a half at any one time.

You may find that, after one feeding, your baby is awake for an hour and forty-five minutes; then you need to make up for this loss of sleep by letting him sleep longer after the next feed. If your baby is up for more than two hours, and then only sleeping for half an hour, and then up again at the next feeding, he is being overstimulated.

To ensure proper development, it is crucial for your baby to develop good sleeping skills in the first few months. Your baby's sleep patterns will lay the foundation for how he will sleep through his life. How many times have you heard someone say, "I was never a good sleeper as a child and I'm still not!"

Your new baby's brain is on overdrive, and it requires enough good-quality sleep to develop to its full potential. In addition, a baby dreams when she is sleeping; new research by French neuroscientist Michel Jouvet has shown that infants' brains respond to exercise, excitement, and dreaming (in REM sleep), stimulating neuronal connections and other growth factors. Unfortunately, poor sleep in infancy has been linked to less than optimal brain and body development, and other negative health conditions later in life, including childhood and adult obesity.

If your baby is awake for more than an hour and a half at a time, then it's possible you are missing her cues and keeping her up too long. If you think this is the case, then try putting her down a little sooner. I have seen a few moms so desperate for a night's sleep that they have tried to keep their baby awake all day, only to then have a restless night. The more tired your baby gets, unfortunately the less she will sleep and the harder it will be for her to settle.

One little girl I took care of was a serious sleeper: she awakened at 7:00 A.M. and was happy to be awake for exactly one and a half hours. Then, presto! Like a Cinderella's magic coach, she turned right into a pumpkin at 8:30 A.M. and had to go to sleep. I would wake her for her 10:00 A.M. bottle, and she would go straight back to sleep until her bottle at 1:00 P.M. After the 1:00 P.M. feeding, she had more of an awake period again. But she absolutely loved her morning nap. Her afternoon nap was only an hour, since she slept so well the rest of the time. And because of these good naps she was getting in the early part of the day, she slept much more easily at night. On the occasional day when she was a little irritated with gas and hadn't slept so peacefully through the day, she tended to have a more restless night; but once her tummy issues were settled, she went right back to her old good habits. So, if your baby has an off day with some gas or tummy problems, don't worry—everything will probably be better tomorrow.

You should now be able to put your baby down in her bassinet/crib and have her go to sleep on her own. So when your baby is ready to sleep, change her diaper, swaddle her, hug her and kiss her, and then rock her for just a little while, then gently lay her down. Occasionally she may need you to pat and shush her a little, but if you have been consistent with putting her down to sleep semi-awake, she should now be comfortable with the routine.

The only things that will stop your baby from

drifting off to sleep at this time are a little gas or a burp if he didn't get them all out. You will notice when this happens because your baby will try to settle and then start to squirm a little until he either releases the gas or needs your help to get rid of the burp. So, when he starts to squirm, don't go running to him; if he can take care of it himself, that is great and then he will resettle. If it's a burp, he may not be able to resettle himself; he may need you to pick him up until he has burped and then you can gently place him back in his bed again.

SCHEDULE TROUBLESHOOTING

What could be some of the issues you may be having right now that make this schedule not flow as smoothly as I make it sound? Here are some questions that moms commonly ask me during Week Five:

1. **HOW DO I KNOW WHEN IT'S NAPTIME?**
    Observe your baby and watch for the little telltale signs: yawning, loss of interest in you or toys, or a glazed look on his face.

2. MY BABY ALWAYS WAKES UP AFTER HALF AN HOUR; WHAT DO I DO?

Don't let your baby dictate the sleep time—you're the teacher. Encourage your baby to go back to sleep. Pick her up and gently rock her almost back to sleep, then pat and shush until she settles. Consistently doing this will teach your baby to sleep longer. Occasionally, your baby may have been woken by a burp that got trapped, so help her release the burp, then settle her back down to sleep. Just because she has woken from her nap, that does not mean she is done with her nap.

3. WHAT DO I DO IF MY BABY IS STILL ASLEEP AT 7:00 A.M.?

I recommend waking him very slowly by unswaddling his blanket, turning on the lights, opening the shades, talking to him, and letting him stretch. This can take up to 10 minutes. Then, get him up, change his diaper, and start his day with a feeding. It's better to encourage the wake-up time in order to let the rest of the day flow easier. Your baby won't suffer or be uncomfortable, and will actually begin to enjoy this little waking ritual.

Also, by not taking him out of bed straight away and teaching him to wake to such a calm, comforting routine, you are allowing him to learn to wake happily and not to start to cry out for you immediately. You will eventually have an older baby who wakes happily and is content to stretch and babble and wait until you come to him, instead of a baby who has learned to wake up and cry to get your attention.

4. MY BABY WAS AWAKE AT 5:00 A.M. AND DIDN'T GO BACK TO SLEEP TILL 6:00 A.M. DO I STILL WAKE HER AT 7:00 A.M.?

The answer is yes, you do still wake her. This will probably mean she won't have such a long awake time after the 7:00 A.M. feeding, as she will be a little sleepier. That is fine. Go right back to your regular schedule.

5. MY BABY IS VERY FUSSY IN THE EVENING AND WON'T SETTLE; WHAT CAN I DO?

This is quite common around Week Five. Babies often go through the witching hour in the earlier part of the evening, and so they have a harder time settling down to sleep. When this happens, your baby may need a little more comforting. So, after his bath, feeding, diaper change, and swaddle, he should be put down to bed. If he is resisting this, you may need to pick him up and rock him a little to get him relaxed and then put him down again semi-awake. Pat his side gently and shush until he settles himself down to sleep. Sometimes you will have to repeat this process a few times before he will settle.

I cannot emphasize enough your role as guide. While other philosophies propose that you go with your baby's natural rhythm and put them down only when they are ready to sleep, I strongly disagree. Your baby is not old enough or mature enough to self-regulate. She is looking to her caregiver (you!) to regulate her, especially in these early weeks and months.

In addition, most of us have to work. We have to shop, prepare food, bathe, and participate in all the normal daily motions in our life. When your baby is on her routine, you know you have time to make some food, take a bath, have a nap, spend some time with your husband, watch a little TV—or just have a little time for yourself. Believe me, you will be a much better parent and you will enjoy the wake time you have with your little one so much more!

Note: Most babies don't catch their first cold, or get sick, until they are several months old, though it can happen. If your baby is ill, don't try to maintain the eating and sleeping schedule. Once the baby is well again, you get them back on schedule as soon as it is practical.

WHAT'S GOING ON WITH YOUR BABY: WEEK FIVE

● ● ● ● ● ●

CRADLE CAP

At Week Five, some babies develop what is called *cradle cap*, a form of dermatitis caused by overproduction of oil from the oil glands. Babies' bodies often have a difficult time regulating the production of oil.

You may notice that your baby has developed a flaky, or sometimes even crusty, layer on his head or in his hair. This flakiness can also appear on the eyebrows. In very severe cases, you may even notice it on his back and sometimes even on his chest. Cradle cap is very common; in most cases, it is easily treated and is not a cause for concern. However, you should let your pediatrician know what is going on.

For a mild case of cradle cap, I have found that the best solution is to use olive oil. Simply rub a little olive oil into the flaky area. It's okay to rub it on his head and forehead. Leave it on for about an hour. (True, baby won't look quite so cute with an oily head, and you should put a protective sheet down if you lay him down during this time.) Then gently wash the hair with baby shampoo, using a soft brush and moving in little, circular motions; this will help lift the flaky skin. You don't want to rub so hard that you scrape the skin off and leave the head sore, but you don't want to be too gentle that you fail to remove the flakes. You need do this only once a day; stop as soon as you see an improvement, which usually comes with only a couple of treatments.

The olive oil used to treat the cradle cap doesn't actually stop the cradle cap; it merely helps to remove the crusty dry skin that is caused by the cradle cap. Even though the condition is caused by overproduction of oil, it actually creates a really dry crusty layer of skin. The oil simply removes it in a safe way. If a parent were to try to pick at these dry crusts, it could cause open sores or wounds, leaving the exposed area susceptible to infection.

With more severe cases of cradle cap, I have used a mixture of licorice root drops (purchased from a health food store) and calendula cream (my favorite brand is California Baby). Take a quarter-size dollop of calendula cream and add six drops of licorice root; mix them and rub onto your baby's head. Leave the mixture on your baby's skin for an hour, then wash your baby's head with a gentle shampoo. Again, you should see a drastic improvement in just a couple of days.

Your pediatrician may recommend using a dandruff shampoo, which can also address the issue. However, in my experience, the calendula cream and licorice root drops are gentler on the baby's skin and often more effective, more quickly. Ultimately, the best way to prevent cradle cap is always to use a soft brush at bath time; as you shampoo your baby's hair, gently brush it in a circular motion at each wash. I always do this with the babies I work with, and only once did I come across a baby with cradle cap. Coincidently, this was the one and only time the mom didn't think it was necessary to use the brush when shampooing the baby's hair.

HICCUPS

Hiccups are a contraction of the baby's diaphragm, a portion of muscle and connective tissue that separates the chest and abdominal cavities. Your baby has probably been having hiccups since before she was born, but it may seem to be happening more frequently now.

There is no way to prevent hiccups, or even to stop them, for a matter of fact. Hiccups usually occur after feeding, and in particular after burping. Sometimes a little extra milk will help take the hiccups away, but not always. Sometimes your baby can get hiccups if she gets a little cold, so you may need to check the temperature and add a layer of clothing. Hiccups look much worse to us than they really feel to your baby. The only time you should worry about hiccups is when they prevent your baby from eating or sleeping.

MISSHAPEN HEAD SYNDROME

Plagiocephaly, or misshapen head syndrome, has become much more of an issue now that it is recommended that all babies to sleep on their backs as a way to help prevent sudden infant death syndrome (SIDS). Because their skulls are soft and pliable when they're born, a baby's head can develop a flat spot, owing to pressure on that area when sleeping. When your baby lies in the same spot to sleep, it puts pressure on that part of the skull.

Many vaginally delivered babies are born with an oddly shaped head, caused by the pressure of passing through the birth canal. This usually corrects itself within about six weeks. But if your baby's head hasn't rounded out by six weeks—or if you first notice that your baby has a flat spot on her skull after six weeks of age—it's probably a case of positional plagiocephaly.

This situation shows up most often in babies who are reported to be "good sleepers," babies with unusually large heads, and babies who are born prematurely and have weak muscle tone. The best way to help avoid a misshapen head is to switch the position of your baby's head each time you put him down to sleep. That is, alternate between putting your baby's head turned to the left and to the right each time, and sometimes flat on the back. Also, when you have your baby on the floor for playtime, encourage him to move his head from side to side, so that it doesn't stay in one place.

Babies with torticollis can also develop a flat spot on their skulls because they often sleep with their heads turned to one side. Torticollis occurs when a tight or shortened muscle on one side of the neck causes the chin to tilt to the other side. Premature babies are especially prone to torticollis. If you notice your baby's head is always tilted to one side, you should definitely discuss this with your pediatrician. You will probably be given a set of exercises to do with your baby to help correct the torticollis. This condition can come and go over a period of months, so don't automatically assume that once it looks better, it won't come back.

ENGAGE YOUR BABY

NURSERY RHYMES

If you've followed my advice, you've already been talking, singing, and reading to your baby. But for some reason, Week Five is a great time to introduce nursery rhymes. If you have recordings of nursery rhymes to play for baby, then do so now, as he will enjoy the rhythm and the interaction with you. Using little hand movements to go along with the rhymes can really stimulate your baby. You can also use a hand puppet or finger puppet to talk to your baby in a high, sing-song voice.

GRASPING REFLEX: IT'S RATTLE TIME!

Your baby is now beginning to develop her grasping technique, so this is a good time to let her play with some little rattles or rings. This provides tactile stimulation as well as encourages hand-eye coordination.

MOVE AROUND, SEE THE WORLD

Your baby will love having a tour of your house. Many babies I have worked with have enjoyed looking at pictures and paintings in their homes. Sometimes they just love to look out the window and stare at a tree. Watch to see what objects interest your baby and point them out and talk about the objects.

When you do your routine chores around the house, keep your baby close and describe your activities or sing while doing them. Your baby will love being carried around in a sling or wrap. But remember—when it is naptime, it's always best to swaddle her and put her down in her bassinet, crib, or stroller.

WHAT ABOUT *YOU?*

. . . . . .

By Week Five, you should be well on the way to feeling completely healed from an episiotomy or c-section procedure. You shouldn't be feeling any serious discomfort, so if you do still feel some pain, you should contact your doctor just to make sure everything is okay, even if you've already scheduled your own six-week checkup with your Ob-Gyn.

Your emotions may still be all over the place. My motto is, Just let it out! It's so much better than trying to be the martyr and hold it in. In the months to come, you can have a good laugh about the things you cry about now. For instance, you may find it hard to watch sad or scary or frightening shows (like the TV news, sometimes), so best to avoid it. Take care and enjoy every moment of this precious time. You'll have plenty of time to catch up when your baby is a little bigger.

IF YOU'RE FEELING QUITE BLUE, DEPRESSED, OR ANXIOUS

Your baby is just so perfect in every way, and everyone is so happy for you. Everyone, that is, except you. If this is supposed to be such a happy time, why do

you feel so low? Some degree of emotional vulner-
ability is natural and expected after childbirth. In
general, these feelings of being overwhelmed last no
longer than two weeks. If you have the blues, you may
be weepy, anxious, and unable to sleep. You may also
be irritable or moody. Moms often feel better after
getting some rest and a helping hand with the baby.
But if your feelings have lasted more than two weeks,
it may be the start of postpartum depression.

Postpartum depression (PPD) is a serious mood
disorder that can harm you, your baby, and the rest of
your family. It can begin any time during the first two
months, and its symptoms typically include:

- Irritability or hypersensitivity
- Difficulty concentrating
- Anxiety and worry
- Crying or tearfulness
- Anger
- Negative feelings, such as sadness,
  hopelessness, helplessness, or guilt
- Loss of interest in activities you usually enjoy
- Difficulty sleeping (especially in returning to
  sleep)
- Fatigue or exhaustion
- Changes in appetite or eating habits

- Headaches, stomachaches, muscle-aches or backaches

Some women with PPD believe they can't actually cope with the care of their baby or, worse, may feel they may harm their baby. As PPD can also be accompanied by extreme anxiety and even panic, some women experience both depression and anxiety, whereas others describe feeling either depressed or anxious. Here is a list of symptoms:

- Extreme anxiety or irritability
- Restlessness and agitation
- Shortness of breath
- Chest pains or discomfort
- Sensation of choking or smothering
- Dizziness
- Tingling in hands or feet
- Trembling and shaking
- Sweating
- Faintness
- Hot or cold flashes
- Fear of dying, of going crazy, or of losing control

Some women with postpartum anxiety have recurrent fears about harm coming to their children, other loved ones, or themselves. Doctors think that some women are more likely than others to get post-partum depression if they, or other family members, have a history of anxiety or depression.

Although current issues, such as a difficult preg-nancy or childbirth, marital stress, or loss of a loved one can trigger PPD, these circumstances don't actu-ally cause the condition. However, if you feel any of the symptoms described here, seek professional help, counseling, and medication. Ask your primary care physician or Ob-Gyn for a recommendation or referral.

Counseling is good, as it may help a mom to talk through her concerns with a psychiatrist, psy-chologist, or other mental health professional. The counseling will help you to learn better ways to cope with your feelings and solve problems, while setting realistic goals. You may also ask for help with fam-ily or relationship issues, as these can sometimes be related to PPD. Antidepressants are a proven ther-apy for PPD. However, if you are breast-feeding, it's important to let your doctor know; most medica-tions will enter the breast milk. There are some anti-depressants that can be used while breast-feeding. Hormone therapy may also help with PPD. In addi-tion, estrogen replacement can help counteract the rapid drop in estrogen levels after childbirth and may erase or ease the symptoms of PPD for some women.

Unfortunately, moms with postpartum depression often have trouble falling and/or staying asleep. If this is the case, try to simply take a rest, even if you just read a magazine or watch TV. Ask a relative or friend to watch your baby for an hour or so each day. If you don't have family or friends around, consider hiring someone who has experience with newborns.

Here are some recommendations I make regardless of whether or not you have a PPD diagnosis:

• Take care of yourself! It's so important for moms to make sure their own basic needs are met, which comes down to getting enough rest, sleep, and food. This also means taking time each day to take a shower, go for a walk, or do some other nonintense exercise.

• Don't expect so much of yourself. Right now, it is enough just to get out of bed and face the day. If you can focus on taking good care of yourself, you'll be doing well.

• Part of being a good mother is knowing when to ask for help, so don't be afraid to ask for it during this difficult time. Help comes in many forms, ranging from friends who cook meals and fold your laundry to therapy. You need support from others so you can get better.

• Reach out to your husband, or partner, or a friend, or someone you trust about how you feel.

• Join a mommy group. Most communities offer ways for new moms, or moms with new babies, to get together and trade information. No one is more sympathetic than another woman going through exactly what you are going through!

• Spend time outside. If the weather permits, put your baby in a stroller and take a walk around the block, or meet a friend at a nearby park, library, or coffee shop. The fresh air, sunshine, and conversation will do you and your baby a world of good. If even a brief excursion is too much for you right now, then just go outside, close your eyes, take a deep breath, and sit in the sunshine for a few minutes. It will help.

• Relax. If you can't keep your house or apartment up to your strict standards of cleanliness, give yourself a break.

Remember, just because you have PPD, that doesn't mean you are a bad mother or don't love your child. Once you get help and feel better, these feelings will disappear.

Week Five does not have to be hell week. In fact, if you review some of my advice for the early few weeks, you can avoid or offset some of the triggers for sleep deprivation, emotional moodiness, and even the blues that might otherwise come at this point. The key is this: taking the best care of your baby means taking the best care of *you*. The two go hand in hand, now more than ever before in your life.

CHAPTER 9

WEEK SIX.
PROUD PARENTS TELL ALL:
A BABY CAN LEARN TO SLEEP
THROUGH THE NIGHT

How many times have you heard new moms ask one another, "Is your baby sleeping through the night?" Hundreds, probably. Have you cringed in worry? Ducked your head, not wanting the question to be asked of you?

Well, cringe no more. This is the week you are going to become one of those moms who can turn to her friends and say, "My baby is sleeping through the night." Hooray!

But before you jump up and down with excitement or fall over in relief, let's first talk about what "sleeping through the night" really means. The true definition of a baby's sleeping through the night at six weeks is a baby who will sleep six to eight hours straight. So, if your baby takes his Dream Feed at 10:00 P.M., and the rest of the day and evening schedule is consistent (as described in Weeks One to Five), then your baby should now be sleeping until 4:00 to 6:00 A.M. I know, waking up at 4:00 A.M. is not your ideal morning call, but when a baby sleeps from 10:00 P.M. to 4:00 A.M. or from 10:00 P.M. to 5:00 A.M., that means you can (and should) sleep straight through those times, too. If you do, you will no longer have that overwhelming feeling that comes from having your deep sleep interrupted two or three times a night. Instead, your body and brain will rest for seven to eight hours, which will make you feel absolutely human again!

It's important to keep in mind that sleeping from 7:00 P.M. to 7:00 A.M. doesn't happen until your baby reaches about four months. Many moms and dads drive themselves crazy thinking that their baby should be sleeping through the night much earlier, when physically a baby cannot do more than a seven- or eight-hour stretch of sleep without needing to eat. Their nervous systems have to mature, and their tummies have to get a little bigger before they can go the full night.

Our goal in Week Six is to set up your baby to do

a nice, long stretch from the Dream Feed to the early hours of the morning. But before you begin to worry or wonder if that is truly possible, take a deep breath and let's go over a few ground rules.

WEEK SIX SCHEDULE

Y ou should be finding your baby is settling into this schedule easily now, whether you are breast-feeding or bottle-feeding.

7:00 A.M.	Feeding
7:30 A.M.	Playtime
8:30 A.M.	Naptime
10:00 A.M.	Feeding
11:00 A.M.	Naptime
1:00 P.M.	Feeding
1:30 P.M.	Playtime
2:30 P.M.	Naptime
4:00 P.M.	Feeding
4:30 P.M.	Playtime
5:00–5:30 P.M.	Naptime
6:45 P.M.	Bath time
7:00 P.M.	Feeding

7:30 P.M.	Bedtime
10:00 P.M.	Dream Feed
5:00 A.M.	Feeding
7:00 A.M.	Feeding

Again, use this schedule as a guide and adjust as needed. Some babies will sleep a little more and some a little less. But you want to try to stay close to this routine and not let your baby have too much awake time, lest she get restless and be unable to settle into the sleep she needs.

THE FLOW OF WEEK SIX

● ● ● ● ● ●

Week Six is the time to make sure the nighttime routine is well established and in place. The nighttime routine starts with the bath, then getting dressed for sleeping.

Bath time at this point should still be every other night, but you can introduce baby lotion so your baby's skin doesn't get too dry. While you are getting your baby dressed for bed, play his calm, relaxing music. One family I worked for put together their selection of music on an iPod, then asked if they could shuffle the play list. You don't want to do this; it's the consistency of the music that gives your baby the cue that it's time for sleep.

SCHEDULE TROUBLESHOOTING

Parents do complain about waking their baby at 7:00 A.M. when she has just had a feeding at 5:00 A.M. They'd rather go back to sleep themselves, and they don't think it's necessary to wake up the baby for that feeding at 7:00 A.M. But this is not the case: if you start your baby's day later, then her day will end later.

When I first started working as a baby nurse, I worked for one mom who insisted on keeping her baby asleep until 9:00 A.M. I didn't complain at the time; I was happy to get a little extra sleep myself (after all, I was the one up the most at night!). But soon her baby wouldn't settle for the night until 9:00 or 10:00 P.M. This is different from the 10:00 P.M. Dream Feed because, if your baby isn't asleep, then you're not lifting her in a sleepy state to feed. It was the equivalent of giving your baby the 7:00 P.M. going-to-bed feeding.

Managing Multiples

How does this routine work for multiples? Pretty much the same. If you have twins, always encourage the first one who wakes up to sleep a little longer by patting and shushing; when the second baby wakes up, go ahead and feed them both. However, if both your babies are waking early, you will need to encourage both to settle back down. I always like to set myself a specific time goal for the sleep. I encourage the babies to sleep to this time for three nights, and then I start pushing for longer. If you don't reach the time goal the first night, don't worry; just keep pushing toward it. If you are consistent about patting and shushing until your babies are almost asleep, they will quickly learn to resettle themselves.

It obviously is a little trickier with triplets, but the same principles can work. It's all about teaching your babies to settle themselves. I have worked with triplets and have been very successful in getting them to sleep for the same time period . . . So, if one baby stirs, resettle him until the second baby wakens. At this point, feed the two of them and allow the third to sleep. As soon as the two have finished eating, feed the third baby—unless that baby is totally asleep. If that's the case, I might be tempted to let him sleep, just to see how long he would go. Then, the next night I would try to hold off the first two who woke earlier the night before, so they could learn to sleep as long as the third baby. However, don't make yourself crazy—if they really won't settle, go ahead and feed.

If I tried to put the baby down sooner, he fussed and complained, and sometimes just screamed. His witching hour was at 8:00 or 9:00 P.M., and there was no getting around it. This ultimately upset his whole schedule because he was always overtired and not getting the rest when he needed it. I tried talking the mom into getting her baby's day started earlier, but she wouldn't listen to me. Six months after I left the family, I got a call from the mom, who asked if there was anything I could do to help, as now her baby wouldn't go to sleep until 10:30 at night and slept until 9:30 or 10:00 in the morning.

"That's the problem," I told her as gently as possible. At eight months, a baby will happily sleep eleven or twelve hours at night, but if he is sleeping until 9:00 or 10:00 in the morning, he certainly is not going to be sleepy until 10:00 or 11:00 at night.

Of course, setting your baby's schedule is entirely up to you. It really is nice to tuck your little one into bed and then still be able to enjoy a little time with your partner, instead of dropping down exhausted! One day your little baby will have to go to school, and school starts a lot earlier than 10:00 A.M. It is easy to adjust your child's schedule as a baby, but much harder as he gets older.

It's the *consistency* of the routine you have established for your baby that makes the whole sleeping schedule work. So, if your baby wakes at 4:00 or 5:00 A.M., and is (more than likely) hungry, let her eat until she is falling back asleep. With some babies, this may be a small amount of 2 ounces; if you have a hungrier baby, this could be a full feeding of 4 ounces. Then, at 7:00 A.M., feed her again, knowing she will probably eat a little less than usual. Ideally, the goal is to give the baby a little less at 4:00 or 5:00 A.M. then let her have a full feeding at 7:00 A.M.

If your baby wakes at 6:00 A.M. or later, then it's a little trickier to stick to your schedule because most babies won't be interested in a feeding only an hour later. In this case, try to hold your baby off as long as possible before you feed him, pushing as close to 7:00 A.M. as possible, by trying to resettle him or just having a little interaction time. You can try talking to your baby or giving him that little stretch and wake up time in his bassinet, and taking your time with changing the diaper.

If your baby keeps waking up very hungry at 6:00 A.M., then try adjusting the daytime feedings by five or ten minutes throughout the day to get back on track. Sometimes, you don't even have to stretch them to the 10:00 A.M. feeding; the baby will go that long all on his own. But if he doesn't, adjust the schedule a little each feeding as needed.

However, all babies' temperaments are different, and if you have a child who won't be held off, then go ahead and feed your baby; but you may need to give him another little feeding at 7:30 A.M. to get him back on schedule for the 10:00 A.M. feeding. Again, you may have to adjust the feedings by five or ten minutes throughout the day to get back on track.

I always try to push for the first option, as it then helps encourage a baby to be content while waiting a little and not always be demanding things straight away. Teaching your baby that she can wait will ultimately help her as she learns to self-soothe and become an independent sleeper, which are both very important parts of her development.

A QUICK REVIEW: PROMOTING GOOD SLEEP HABITS _____

1. IS YOUR BABY SWADDLED AND SECURE?

I so often hear a parent say to me, "My baby doesn't like being swaddled, and she is always fighting to get out." Just because your baby gets her arms out of a swaddle doesn't mean she doesn't like it. When you go to sleep at night, do you wake up in exactly the same position? Probably not. Babies are the same. They move in their sleep. A lot of the time, they haven't been swaddled firmly enough, and this allows the little movement to undo the swaddle and so the baby breaks out.

You still want to swaddle your baby because, since a baby's nervous system isn't fully developed yet, she will twitch much more out of the swaddle—which will more often than not result in waking up prematurely. The phrase "sleeping like a baby" doesn't come from how long a baby sleeps; it is based on a baby's ability to sleep where and whenever she is tired. Who hasn't seen a baby propped on a shopping cart in what looks like the most uncomfortable position—fast asleep! Or, when a baby falls asleep in the car seat with her head dropped forward? Can you imagine the pain we would have in our necks when we woke up from that?

2. IS YOUR BABY WARM ENOUGH OR TOO HOT?

Many times parents want to make their baby's room too warm, assuming that babies need to be incubated at a higher temperature. Your baby's room doesn't need to be any warmer than 72 degrees at night. If you live in a cooler climate, then 68 to 70 degrees is warm enough. If you make the room too hot, it can make it hard for your baby to breathe. You also need to dress your baby appropriately. The general rule of thumb is that your baby should have one more layer than you, as babies don't regulate their temperature as well and they don't sleep under a nest of blankets or a comforter. So, if you go to bed with cotton pajamas, then just make sure your baby's pajamas are a little warmer, or maybe put a onesie under his pajamas. Remember, he also has his swaddle blanket, so that gives the extra layer.

3. ARE YOU JUMPING UP AND GOING TO YOUR BABY EVERY TIME SHE MAKES A LITTLE SQUEAK OR NOISE?

This is a very common thing for first-time or anxious parents. Babies make little noises all night long, and it's often hard for parents to not listen to these goos and gurgles. Their breathing can also change a little. This is normal, and shouldn't worry you. Unfortunately, because this often happens when babies are in their light sleep, and you come running to see if she's okay, you usually wake her up, disturbing the sleep cycle.

What to do? Use my Count-to-Ten Rule. If you just can't resist having a peek to make sure your baby is fine, then go in as quietly as possible and try not to let her see you. If you are one of those parents who just can't deal with not being able to see what your baby is doing, then invest in a video monitor. That way, you can look without disturbing your baby.

Note: None of this applies if your baby is crying

hard or screaming. If your baby is crying, then you will need to see what is wrong.

4. **DOES YOUR BABY OFTEN WAKE UP CRYING AT NIGHT?**

This can be happening for a few different reasons. First, is your baby gassy? Have you burped your baby enough before putting him down for the night? The 10:00 P.M. feeding can often be a challenging burping time, as you are feeding your baby in a semi-sleepy state and so by the time you get the burp up, your baby could be falling back to sleep. However, it is better to wake him a little in the burping process to get the burps up than to have him wake a little while later because he is uncomfortable.

Or, is your baby crying for you at night? If he doesn't know how to get back to sleep, he will cry out for your assistance. How should you deal with this? You will need to go to your baby, but *don't* pick your baby up. *Don't* give him a pacifier or any other assistance. Check that he doesn't have a dirty diaper or hasn't spit up. If you need to change his diaper or his clothes, do so in dim light, without talking. Then, quietly tell your baby you are there and everything is okay. Gently pat him on his side until he settles. If he is used to your doing anything else, he won't necessarily be happy with your simply patting him and telling him all is okay, so be prepared when he might get a bit fussy or upset. But being consistent with this routine will pay off in a few short nights, instead of endless sleepless nights!

The most important thing is to stop the patting before your baby goes back to sleep. Remember, you are teaching him to put himself to sleep, even if it takes an hour the first time; I promise you it will get better. Consistency reaps the rewards. Occasionally your baby won't settle like this to begin with, so you will need to pick him up, but only hold him for as long as it takes to settle him, then put him back in his crib and pat and shush a little to keep him settled. But don't pat and shush until he's asleep!

When a Cry Means Something More

Your baby could be crying out at night for health-related issues, including pain from reflux. The good news is that you can help prevent some of this discomfort by tilting your baby's mattress so he sleeps with his head higher than his feet, which helps stop the acid from rising.

If you think your baby may have reflux, consult your doctor right away. It may simply be a case of waiting for your baby's digestive system to mature, or your baby may benefit from medication.

WHAT'S GOING ON WITH YOUR BABY: WEEK SIX

· · · · · ·

At the six week mark, some of your baby's physical, social, and cognitive milestones will come into sight. Did you just hear your baby coo? Is she constantly trying to grab, grab, grab? Your baby is practicing her grip (on your finger or her rattle) and starting to reach for objects as her hand-eye coordination improves every day. This is the second big growth-spurt week. Expect your baby to be a little hungrier, wanting to nurse longer at the breast, or needing more milk in her bottle. This is fine—give her a little more.

Her sensory perception is growing as well; this is a good time to introduce some new objects, such as colorful rubbery toys, small board books, and mirrors. You may also want to ramp up activities that you do with your baby, including playing music and clapping along; dancing around to the music with your baby, or pointing out natural sights if you are outside taking a walk.

It's important to stress tummy time: your baby should be able to lift his head briefly when on his tummy on a flat surface.

But most special of all, it's during Week Six that

most babies give their parents their first smile. Remember to smile back! It's your response that will encourage him to smile more. You should notice that your baby will now turn his head and eyes to look toward a light source or the sound of your voice. If you move an object slowly across your baby's field of vision, he'll track it with his eyes. The eye movements will still be a bit jerky, but the more you offer him an opportunity, the more he will strengthen his eyes.

When she coos, coo back, then stop and let her respond. Sticking your tongue out at her now will signal for her to do the same. This is your baby's first form of imitation, and will encourage her to copy other things that you do. You may feel a bit silly sticking out your tongue at your baby, but rest assured that imitation is a natural way moms support baby learning.

Your baby may not be able to talk yet, but his face is definitely telling you a lot. He's experimenting with different facial expressions—pursing his lips, raising his eyebrows, widening his eyes, or squinting and furrowing his brow. Your baby may recognize and anticipate your breast or a bottle by moving his arms and legs and cooing excitedly.

Even though these are all signs of your baby's emerging development, not all children learn or express these skills at the same time.

UPCOMING DOCTOR VISITS
AND VACCINES

By Week Six, you will want to begin thinking about vaccinations. Your baby is just two weeks away from her two-month checkup, which is typically when most babies start a cycle of six vaccines between birth and six months old. These vaccines will protect your baby from eight serious diseases.

I know that there is some controversy surrounding vaccines. My position is that vaccines prevent diseases that have killed and crippled many, many children and adults. Not vaccinating your child puts him at risk. I believe all children should be vaccinated; the risks of not having the vaccinations far outweigh the small risks of having the vaccinations. According to the American Academy of Pediatrics:

1. In the 1950s, before there was a vaccine, *polio* paralyzed about 37,000 people and killed about 1,700 others each year.
2. In the 1980s, Hib was the leading cause of *bacterial meningitis* in children under the age of five.
3. Before the vaccine was developed, 15,000 people died each year from *diphtheria*.

4. Most children have had at least one *rotovirus* infection by their fifth birthday.

None of these diseases has completely disappeared, and without the vaccinations, they will come back to endanger more children and their families.

The eight diseases prevented by childhood vaccinations are:

1. *Diptheria*, a bacterial infection spread via contact with an infected person. Signs and symptoms include a thick covering in the back of the throat that can make it hard to breathe. It can lead to breathing problems, heart failure, and death.

2. *Tetanus*, a bacterial infection that is picked up from a cut or wound. It is not contagious. Symptoms include painful tightening of the muscles, usually all over the body. It can lead to stiffness of the jaw so that the victim can't open his mouth or swallow. Infection leads to death in about one case in five.

3. *Pertussis,* or whooping cough, is a bacterial infection that is spread via physical contact (touching) with an infected person. Signs and symptoms include violent coughing spells that can make it hard for an infant to eat,

drink, or breathe. These spells can last for
weeks. It can lead to pneumonia, seizures,
brain damage, and death.

4. *Hib*, or influenza type B, is a bacterial
infection passed from person to person
through skin, saliva (coughing), and blood.
There may be no symptoms in mild cases, but
this strain of the flu can lead to meningitis,
pneumonia, and infections of the blood,
joints, bones, and covering of the heart, as
well as brain damage, deafness, and death.

5. *Hepatitis B* is a virus transmitted by the blood
or body fluid of an infected person. Babies
can get it at birth if their mother is infected,
or through a cut or wound. Adults can get
it from unprotected sex, sharing needles,
or other exposures to blood. Signs and
symptoms include tiredness, diarrhea and
vomiting, jaundice, and pain in the muscles,
joints, and stomach. It can lead to liver
damage, liver cancer, and death.

6. *Polio* is a virus transmitted by close contact
with an infected person. It enters through
the mouth. Signs and symptoms can include
a coldlike illness, or there may be no signs
or symptoms at all. It can lead to paralysis or
death.

7. *Pneumococcal pneumonia* (inflammation of the lung) is caused by an infection by a number of infectious agents, including bacteria, viruses, fungi, and parasites. Symptoms include fever, chills, cough, and chest pain. It can lead to meningitis, blood infections, pneumonia, deafness, brain damage, and death.

9. *Rotovirus* is a virus that spreads via hand-to-mouth contact, even if the infected person doesn't have symptoms. Symptoms in children include severe diarrhea, vomiting, and fever. It can lead to severe dehydration requiring hospitalization and, in severe cases, death. Adults can show mild or no symptoms.

How Vaccines Work

Vaccines are made with the same bacteria or viruses that cause the specific diseases, but they have been weakened or killed to make them safe. A child's immune system responds to the vaccines the same way it would if the child had mild forms of these disease: by creating antibodies that attack the bacteria or viruses. If the child is later exposed to those diseases, the antibodies to fight them are already in place.

RECOMMENDED IMMUNIZATIONS

Here is list of vaccinations recommended by the American Academy of Pediatrics.

1. *DTaP,* to protect against diphtheria, tetanus, and pertussis.
   - At 2 months
   - At 4 months
   - At 6 months
   - Between 15 and 18 months (can be given as early as 12 months as long as it's at least 6 months after the previous shot)
   - Between 4 and 6 years old
   - A booster shot at 11 or 12 years of age

2. *Hepatitis A,* to protect against hepatitis A, which can cause the liver disease hepatitis.
   - Between 12 and 23 months, two shots, with the second given 6 to 18 months after the first

3. *Hepatitis B.*
   - At birth
   - Between 1 and 2 months
   - Between 6 and 18 months

4. *Hib.*
   - At 2 months
   - At 4 months
   - At 6 months (not needed if the PedvaxHIB
     or ComVax brand of vaccine was given at
     2 and 4 months)
   - Between 12 and 15 months

5. *HPV,* to protect against human papillomavirus,
   the most common sexually transmitted disease in
   the United States and a cause of genital warts and
   of cervical, anal, and throat cancers.
   - Three doses for girls and boys at 11 or 12 years
     of age

6. *Influenza* (the flu shot or, for age 2 and up, nasal
   spray vaccine), to protect against seasonal flu and
   H1N1 (swine flu).
   - Age 6 months and up; every year in the fall or
     early winter
   - One dose for most children
   - Two doses for children 6 months to 8 years old
     who are getting the flu vaccine for the first time
     or who had only one dose of the flu vaccine in
     the previous year's flu season

7. *Meningococcal,* to protect against meningococcal disease, previously a leading cause of bacterial meningitis in US children.
   • Between 11 and 12 years

8. *MMR,* to protect against measles, mumps, and rubella (German measles).
   • Between 12 and 15 months
   • Between 4 and 6 years old

9. *Pneumococcal (PCV).*
   • At 2 months
   • At 4 months
   • At 6 months
   • Between 12 and 15 months

10. *Polio (IPV).*
    • At 2 months
    • At 4 months
    • Between 6 and 18 months
    • Between 4 and 6 years old

11. *Rotovirus* (given orally, not as an injection).
    • At 2 months
    • At 4 months
    • At 6 months (not needed if the Rotarix brand of vaccine was given at 2 and 4 months)

12. *Varicella,* to protect against chicken pox.
- Between 12 and 15 months
- Between 4 and 6 years

Scheduling the Vaccinations

When my daughter was an infant, I asked my daughter's pediatrician to spread out her vaccines a little more than the usual schedules suggest. That was eleven years ago. This has now become more of an issue with many pediatricians because of some suggestions that the vaccines are linked to a rising incidence of autism. (These suspicions have proven to be false or misleading by all scientific and medical studies.) However, I have noticed that doctors are more often insisting that babies have their shots when they are due to be given. This really is something you should discuss with your pediatrician. It's important to know whether your pediatrician is happy to give the shots on a more staggered schedule or if his policy is to do them as suggested above. You should be comfortable with what your pediatrician recommends.

If Your Baby Is Sick at the Time

If your child is sick on the day she is due to get vaccinated, you should discuss postponing the vaccination. A baby needs all of her immune-system strength to respond optimally to the vaccine. A child with a mild cold or a low fever can usually be vaccinated that day. But for a more serious vaccination, it is recommended to wait until your child is healthy.

Also, if your child has any life-threatening allergies, reactions to antibiotics or to yeast, or has a weakened immune system, you should talk to your doctor before giving your child any vaccines.

LET'S GET BACK TO *YOU*

N ow that your baby is doing so well, you may have some time to realize that you need a little attention yourself! Just as your body has taken a toll, you may be noticing that your skin has lost that rosy mom-to-be glow. The glow was caused by estrogen-fueled blood flow to your skin, and it may now be replaced with postpartum acne. This is due to hormonal swings, stress, sleep deprivation, and very little time for skin care.

You may also have some dark patches on your forehead, upper lip, and cheeks, and you may be wondering how you can make them disappear. In most cases, these patches—known as the pregnancy mask—are caused by an increase in melanin, a skin pigment, during pregnancy. The good news is that your skin should start slowing down in making so much melanin, although sometimes this won't happen until you wean your baby. Then, the patches will fade and disappear.

You can help the process along by staying out of the sun as much as possible, and always wearing a broad-spectrum sunscreen, rain or shine. Remember: once you have had these dark patches, they are more likely to return. Also, if you go back on the pill, you may want to ask for an estrogen-free variety, as estrogen can sometimes make this condition worse.

Now that you are probably losing more of your baby weight, you may also be noticing your stretch marks. Most women get at least a few stretch marks, but the good news is that they will fade. There are several things you can do to help this along. For example, exercise will help tremendously—but start slowly. Eating right is important, too: stay away from white sugar, refined white carbs, and high-fat foods.

If you continue to eat a healthy, well-rounded diet that emphasizes whole grains, fruits and veggies, and lean protein, you will help your body trim down and your skin replenish itself. Taking a fish oil supplement will also help rebuild the skin. Moisturize regularly (it won't eliminate your stretch marks, but it'll keep itching to a minimum as your tummy gets back in shape). You can also use the Egyptian Magic on your strech marks. It's good for more than diaper rash! One more thing to keep in mind: your baby thinks you're beautiful—stretch marks, freckles, and all!

The other thing you could be noticing now is hair loss. Though your brush says otherwise, postpartum hair loss is not as bad as you think. Many women find that their hair falls out—sometimes in huge amounts—after having a baby. But before you start to worry that there's more hair on your brush than on your head, know that you're not going bald; you're just catching up on normal hair loss. In fact, it's normal for 85 to 95 percent of the hair on your head to be growing while the remainder is in a resting period. After the rest cycle, this hair falls out (typically while you're brushing or shampooing) and is replaced by new growth. The average head sheds 100 hairs a day—just not all at once, so you don't usually notice them. During pregnancy, your hormones prolonged the growing stage (increased estrogen is the reason behind that extra-thick hair), so there are fewer hairs in the resting stage and fewer hairs falling out.

But all good things must come to an end, and fall out they must. So expect all that hair that hung around for the past nine months to shed sometime after delivery (usually between three and six months postpartum). But take comfort knowing that by the time your baby is ready to blow out the candles on her first birthday cake (and has a full head of hair of her own), your hair should be back to normal, too. Remember, not all moms experience dramatic hair changes during pregnancy or after delivery. But for those who do, expect the gains (and losses) to be more obvious if you've got longer hair. Talk to your practitioner if your hair loss seems really excessive. That could be a sign, along with other symptoms, of postpartum thyroiditis, an inflammation of the thyroid gland that can lead to a long-term underactive thyroid.

When you have reached this point, you should be proud of your accomplishments. Your hard work has paid off, and your baby is sleeping nicely. When you tell your friends how well your baby is sleeping, don't let them convince you that you are lucky. I hear this so many times, and it drives me a bit crazy! *It wasn't just luck!* Let your friends know that you taught your baby to sleep, and they can do it, too.

IF YOU JUST FOUND THIS BOOK . . .

If your baby is already six weeks old and you have just picked up this book, it really isn't too late to make changes. Depending on what your baby is doing at this point, it is now a case of putting her on a schedule. As with Week One, the first two things you want to establish is the Dream Feed at 10:00 P.M. and the start of your baby's day at 7:00 A.M. Then, you work toward the three-hour schedule throughout the day.

The other really important matter to work on is how you put your baby to sleep. If you have been using a pacifier, or holding and rocking your baby to sleep, all that needs to stop now. When I took care of a set of triplets who had been using pacifiers, we took them away at about five weeks old. We did it one baby at a time, choosing the one who was less reliant on the pacifier first. Each baby took a few days, and none of them was happy about the change in routine. But ultimately, they slept much better for it. All three soon learned to sleep peacefully, as opposed to the constant waking that occurred when the pacifiers fell out of their mouths. By four months old, all three were sleeping from 7:30 P.M. to 7:00 A.M. So trust me—it can be done.

If your baby was born prematurely, this may be his first week home and you're only just beginning with this book. Depending on your baby's weight and adjusted age (if your baby was born prematurely, her *adjusted age* is the age she would be if she had been carried to full term), you may need to begin at an earlier point in the program—at Week One or Week Two, and then speed up the progression as the baby falls into the feeding and sleeping schedule. However, the hospital will have already set a strict feeding and sleeping schedule for your baby; in that way, it will be easy for you to continue this schedule and then adjust it to work with my guidelines.

CHAPTER 10

AFTER SIX WEEKS: SETTING UP THE REST OF YEAR ONE

So—you have gotten through the first six weeks, and you and your baby are doing well. What now? It is more important than ever to follow through with the consistent schedule and gentle encouragement to get your baby sleeping through until 7:00 A.M.

Let's take a look at the upcoming changes you and your baby will go through over the next few months.

THE FLOW OF THE SCHEDULE

• • • • • •

Often what happens after the first six weeks is that you find your baby consistently waking at the 4:00 to 5:00 A.M. period, and it may seem like she just doesn't want to sleep any longer than that! Some moms feel that this isn't so bad, but you don't have to settle for this situation: your baby can make it through the night with a little more guidance.

If you find that your baby seems to have gotten "stuck" at a certain time, you can teach her to sleep a little longer. Don't give her any milk to go back to sleep; use the settling technique of patting and shushing her and picking her up if she starts to cry. She could be stirring consistently at this time every night because this is her light sleep period, and when you get up to feed her, you're actually getting her up unnecessarily. Some babies will be calmer and settle back down easily on their own or with just a little help, and some babies may need a little more encouragement. If you have a baby who does need a little more help, then just be patient. With consistency in encouraging her to settling down and trust that she will learn to settle herself, she will gradually learn to sleep through this wakeful period.

STICKING TO THE DREAM FEED

You may notice your baby is sleepier at the 10:00 P.M. feeding, making the Dream Feed harder and harder to accomplish. This is often the case when I hear a lot of parents asking me if they can give up on the Dream Feed, as their babies seem so sleepy and they don't like to wake them. But it is more important than ever to continue with that gentle waking and feeding at 10:00 P.M. until your baby is sleeping through the night until at least 6:30 or 7:00 A.M.

Once your baby has done this consistently for two weeks, then you can start to eliminate the 10:00 P.M. Dream Feed—but not cold turkey. Do it gradually, over a period of about two weeks, slowly giving your baby less and less milk. For example, if your baby has been drinking 5 ounces at that time, give him 4 ounces for four days in a row. Then, decrease it to 3 ounces for four days in a row, then decrease it to 2 ounces for four days in a row, then stop. There really is no point in waking your baby for just 1 ounce! This gradual transition away from the feeding will make it much easier on you and your baby, and your baby should continue sleeping until 6:30 or 7:00 A.M. without any interruption.

Waking Happy

You should be finding that your baby is starting to wake in the mornings happily and quietly. Stick to your normal routine of unwrapping your baby each morning and allowing her to stretch and look around in her crib while you talk to her and open the curtains, get her bottles ready, or prepare everything for diapering and changing.

The next few months will become so much nicer to wake up to, with your little one cooing and playing happily by herself until you go in to her.

PHYSICAL AND SOCIAL CHANGES

You will be seeing so many changes each month now, as your baby develops and really starts to show his personality. He will be going through many changes as he moves about so much more. One very noticeable difference will be his hair. By three months, you may start to notice your baby's hair thinning at the back and sides. This is due to his head constantly moving about when he is on the floor for playtime and when he is in his crib sleeping. Because a baby's head is the heaviest part of his body right now, all that weight rubs against the surface and the friction gently pulls the hair out.

If your baby has no hair, and many don't, then this won't be such an issue; in fact, you may start to notice a little more growth on the top of your baby's head.

SAY GOOD-BYE TO THE SWADDLE

By four months, you should have a baby who is happily sleeping through the night, from her 7:00 P.M. feeding to her 6:30 or 7:00 A.M. wake-up time. This means that it's time to say good-bye to the swaddle!

Your baby's nervous system has matured enough now that the startle reflex shouldn't bother her and she can happily sleep with her arms out. Again, this should be a gradual transition. I like to do it by swaddling with just one arm out at first. The first night you do this, you may find your baby to be a little more restless than normal. This is to be expected. Try not to go running to your baby if she is just trying to settle herself; just listen to her and see if she is doing okay. Only go to her if she cries and really needs help. Leave her with one arm out for a week.

Next, swaddle her with both arms out. You actually keep her swaddled from below her arms, which will give her a feeling of security. You will probably notice that, as in the first week, she will be a little fussy as she transitions to no swaddle. After a week of this, you can take away the swaddle altogether and put your baby either in a sleep sack or in warm pajamas. I personally prefer the sleep sack, as this gives the warmth of a blanket without using a blanket, but also has a loose feel of being contained, like the swaddle. If you use pajamas, make sure your baby's feet are covered and warm. The only advantage of the sleep sack, is that if you have a very active little one, it may help prevent her from climbing or jumping from the crib. You can use a sleep sack until your baby is two years old.

DAYTIME ACTIVITY

By month four, your baby should be a lot more active during the day.

You should notice him kicking a lot and talking out loud much, much more. He will also more actively try to imitate your mouth actions, blowing little raspberries, sticking his tongue out incessantly, and trying to roll over. A baby will often find it easier to roll from his stomach to his back, but he should be making attempts to roll from his back to his stomach also. If your baby isn't doing this yet, it might mean he needs a little more time on the floor each day to learn, or he just might not have reached that developmental point yet. Continue to gently encourage him by helping him roll from side to side so he gets the feel of the movement.

At this point you should be stretching your baby's daytime feedings. You should have noticed that he isn't so hungry after three hours and will happily wait until nearly four hours, so go ahead and start stretching the feedings to four-hour intervals. You will probably need to give him an extra ounce in each bottle to help him or let him stay a little longer at the breast. By doing this, you will have cut out a whole bottle, so it is time to give him a little more to compensate. With four-hour feedings, your baby's schedule should be:

7:00 A.M.	Awake and feeding; playtime
9:00 A.M.	Naptime
11:00 A.M.	Feeding; playtime
1:00 P.M.	Naptime
3:00 P.M.	Feeding; playtime
5:00 P.M.	Short nap (no more than 45 minutes); playtime
6:30 P.M.	Bath time
7:00 P.M.	Feeding and off to bed

In today's society, parents are under a lot of pressure to do everything right when it comes to their baby's development. But with all the information out there, it can be so confusing to know what the right thing is for your baby's brain development. It is important to learn about the different stages of development your child will go through, but don't miss out on all of the joys of parenting because you are trying to figure out the best way to help make your baby the next Einstein.

You might think that the more you stimulate your baby, the smarter your baby will be, but this isn't necessarily true if you are not creating the right sort of stimulation. The American Academy of Pediatrics recommends that children under the age of two not watch any television, which I agree with wholeheartedly. In fact, TV and videos overstimulate a baby's brain. Learning involves interaction, which your baby cannot get from an electronic device. If you do spend the time interacting with your baby, playing with an electronic toy together, it will be more beneficial than leaving the baby to play (or watch) alone.

Babies need downtime, and it is okay if they experience boredom—parents don't need to constantly worry about keeping babies entertained. In fact, it is during this downtime that children learn how to entertain themselves, creating their own preferences for playing.

The best thing in the world you can do for your baby is to spend quality time with her. For example:

- Talking is the best way to help your baby develop language skills. She will learn from listening to the people around her.
- Laughing and cooing with your baby is a great, interactive experience for both of you. By making your baby laugh, you can learn what he likes or thinks is funny. You will be amazed at the silly things your baby will giggle about. Plus, he will learn by seeing what makes you laugh.
- Cuddling and loving your baby helps her feel secure and wanted, and teaches her how to love. Instead of sitting your baby in front of a screen, cuddle and talk with her.
- Singing to your baby will entertain him, but also expose him to more language. This is a fun way to help your baby develop.
- Reading to your baby will help to stimulate her language development; even though she may not grasp the concept at first, she will eventually. It's good to read books that are cardboard, cloth, or some other textured material (other than paper). This way, your baby can touch and hold the book and you can

point out the pictures, and even sing parts of the story.

- Playing silly games can be so much fun. There is plenty of time in life for you and your baby to be serious, so play silly games together. Not only will your baby have fun, but I bet you will, too. Babies love peekaboo!

There isn't a wrong or right way to parent, as long as there is no abuse or neglect involved. However, I truly believe that you can give your child the best opportunities by spending time, one-on-one with him. Having a new baby is such a big change in anyone's life, even with all the knowledge and experience that's possible. To me, one of the most important ideas to keep in mind always is to enjoy your child, especially her first six weeks, as much as possible. Enjoying this time also means remembering that you are the most perfect person to teach and guide your baby. Without you, your baby has no idea what to do. Contrary to what you may have read in popular magazines, there is no such thing as a manipulative baby. Babies learn what they live and live what they learn. So by laying down a good, firm foundation with good sleeping and eating habits, you should have a happy, contented, delightful baby to enjoy.

ACKNOWLEDGMENTS

I would firstly like to thank Jeff Bernstein for believing in me enough and introducing me to the people who made this book happen.

A huge thank-you to Billie Fitzpatrick, my ghost writer, who has spent hours with me on the phone, through e-mail, and texts helping me to put this book together. Your patience and commitment have been invaluable; without you, this book would not be the same.

To Laura Nolan, my agent, for her great instincts and faith in this book and hard work on my behalf.

To Sydny Miner, my esteemed editor at Crown Books—thank you for looking at the proposal and seeing the potential of this book. I appreciate your patience and support in helping us develop CHERISH to its fullest potential. Thanks, as well, to Anna Thompson, editorial assistant, and all the other knowledgeable, steadfast staff at Crown and Random House, including Mauro DiPreta, Campbell Wharton, Meredith McGinnis, Mary Coyne,

Jim Massey, Elizabeth Rendfleisch, Barbara Sturman, Cathy Hennessy, and Norman Watkins—a huge thank-you to all of you.

To Nicole Kaufman, my illustrator; thank you for the great drawings, which quite simply and brilliantly show what I wanted.

A big thank-you to all the families I have worked with over the years, for all your support and encouragement along the way. And for allowing me to gather the knowledge and experience that has made this book what it is today.

To my best friend, Lynn Katzman, who has always been there to listen to me whenever I needed anything, and helped in anyway possible.

The biggest thank-you goes out to my family, for all your support in the making of this book. To Bryan, for always being so patient and understanding when I needed technical support and someone else's viewpoint. To my two children, who would have sometimes been happier to get out and about, but were understanding when I needed to sit and write this book. To Dad, for always picking up the phone and talking me through all the advice I needed—I love you all!

INDEX